FROM BEER BONGS TO BROCCOLI

The College Kid's Guide To Health and Wellness

ALEXANDRA CATALANO

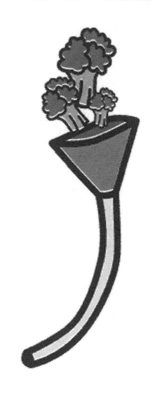

ISBN: 1478107294
ISBN-13: 9781478107293

"If you have health, you probably will be happy,
and if you have health and happiness,
you have all the wealth you need."
—Elbert Hubbard

This book is dedicated to my feisty Italian parents, Frank and Brenda. You may have made me short, but you also made me creative. Ti amo.

Contents

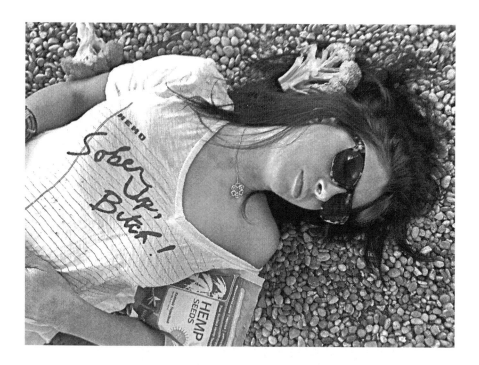

Introduction

So here you are. The day you thought would never come... your first day of college. After all those AP classes, SAT Prep courses, and extracurricular crap, you can finally get what you've been waiting for: freedom! You're finally free of your parents, and you can do whatever you want. You can party all night, dress like a Spice Girl, sleep in class, never clean your room and eat pizza for breakfast. While this experience can be wonderfully liberating, it can also be disastrous for your health if not handled in moderation. We only get one body, and if you don't treat it with the love and care it needs, it can affect the way you look and feel forever.

College is one of the most thrilling times of your life, so why not look and feel your best? It's the one opportunity where you can experience a multitude of new things in a safe and supportive environment. Where else would strangers enthusiastically chant your name while you shotgun a beer? While college provides the perfect setting to discover yourself, many students find themselves experiencing excessive weight gain, low energy, poor skin, frequent illness, depression, and insomnia. Shocking studies conducted by Cornell University found that on average, college freshman gain about 0.5 pounds a week. This is almost 11 times more than the average weight gain among seventeen- and eighteen-year olds and almost 20 times more than the average weight gain among American adults! So we must ask, "Why are college students gaining tremendous amounts of weight so quickly, and how can this be avoided?"

It wasn't long ago that I, too, packed up my room and made my way to college. Finally I had the chance to try new things without the watchful eye of my Italian parents. I didn't know a single person and was excited, yet anxious to begin my new life. College was everything I had hoped it would be and more. However, there was one thing I couldn't help but notice…my expanding waistline. After meeting up with old high school friends during winter break, I realized I wasn't the only one. Apparently there was a name for it: the Freshman 15.

Many of my college friends had put on an exorbitant amount of weight, had poor skin and were so exhausted that they spent most of their day sleeping. When I went home and returned to my original diet, I watched my waistline shrink to its pre-college state, I had more energy, and my skin cleared up. So what was I doing differently? When I returned to college, I began to study my friends', as well as my own personal habits. The first thing I noticed was the food we ate. At home, my Italian mother always prepared fresh, unprocessed, seasonal foods as well as some good old -fashioned Italian Catholic guilt. I ate an abundance of fresh fruits, vegetables, and whole grains—whereas at college, I feasted on frozen pizza, sugary cereals, macaroni and cheese, and drank as much beer as I could stomach before tossing my cookies. I also noticed nobody ever drank water. Glancing around a giant lecture hall, I saw a sea of sodas, coffees, and on occasion, a suspicious flask perhaps containing herbal tea (also known as vodka.) What I rarely saw was students hydrating themselves.

Eating habits were not the only thing that led to my poor health in college. Insufficient sleep, which is often part of the college experience, had a major impact on my overall health and academic performance. In college I was a night owl. I was either up late going to parties, listening to my roommate fight with her long distance boyfriend in Chinese, or glued to my computer writing a paper that was due in two hours. I had pale skin, dark circles under my eyes and was always passing out in class. While living like a vampire was somewhat thrilling, I think we can all agree " The Twilight" thing is on its way out. I had to change and start getting a normal sleep cycle. While I'll admit I've taken the best naps I've ever had during my English 101 class, I realized that my $1,000 dollars a unit class was turning out to be an expensive nap.

Lastly, I found that myself and other students weren't treating the environment with care. Almost every week, my friends and I would throw big parties with unrecyclable red plastic cups, unaware of how many landfills we were contributing to or even considering the colossal waste the university created in general. Think about all the papers, supplies, and books that go unrecycled every semester! The average college student produces an estimated 640 pounds of solid waste each year, including 500 disposable cups and 320 pounds of paper. According to my mathematical calculations that's a shit ton! Each year the numbers continue to grow. So what did I learn in my four years of college?

College is a time of excess. You are constantly pushing the limits to bend all the rules and restrictions that have been instilled in you since your youth. However, four years of constant partying, late night snacks, binge eating, and lack of sleep can do long term damage to your body. It's amazing how much older some students look after their first year of college. They're heavier with wrinkles under their eyes, and lack the energy and zest they once had as bright -eyed freshmen. More importantly, many students carry these poor eating habits into their adult lives and never even consider making a change until it is too late.

After graduating college, you may find yourself in a corporate work environment, where you'll be sedentary at a desk. Either out of boredom or fatigue you might turn to coffee and vendor snacks as a means of nourishment throughout the day. By establishing a balanced diet in your youth, you can continue this healthy life style in the next phase of your life. If you never ate processed foods and drank in excess in college, you would never think of doing that as an adult. Instead of ordering a

Double Whopper for lunch you would be packing fresh fruits, vegetables, whole grains and lean proteins. Then, when you finally get that two-week paid vacation you've been waiting for, you'll look great and have the energy to dance with a hot foreigner with abs like Jesus who speaks broken English or a sassy lady with big jugs! Ole!

As I journeyed from being a college student to a graduate, I found students to be intelligent, compassionate, and talented individuals who possessed tremendous potential to change the world. However, students are not aware of these things because these issues are rarely addressed in college. If students were taught the proper way to love and respect their bodies, they might also begin to show love and respect toward others as well as the environment. I found that when I changed the way I ate, my life started to change as well. My mind became more focused and open to new things, my skin cleared up, I shed extra pounds, I was more productive, and most importantly, I felt more of a connection with others than I ever had in my entire life.

After graduation, I continued my education at the Institute of Integrative Nutrition studying one hundred dietary theories from top experts in the field of health and wellness including Dr. Andrew Weil, David Wolfe, Dr. David Katz, Geneen Roth, Dr. John Douillard, and Dr. Mark Hyman. My goal is to provide the necessary knowledge so that college students are equipped with the tools to be the best they can be.

My intention for writing this book is to help you discover how to give your body the proper love and attention it desperately needs. You will learn how to nourish yourself without counting calories, fad diets, starvation or crying. Instead, I will provide you with a variety of different philosophies and theories to help you achieve optimal health and mental awareness. I will provide the facts, and it will be up to *you* to decide what you choose to embrace. The most important thing you can learn from this book is to understand how to experience something, analyze how you feel, and then determine whether or not your body responds well to it. For example, if you eat dairy and find that you feel bloated after consuming it, you can conclude that dairy should not be a part of your diet. Similarly with alcohol, you can discover that after (x) amount of drinks you get drunk, and after (x) many drinks you become unconscious and do a titty dance on the bar. As a result, you will be able to use this newly gained power to take control of your life and make decisions that will serve you best. You will think with clarity and look and feel great, and it will be a result of choices you made for yourself. There's no better feeling in the world than living in harmony with your values and beliefs.

Many tout college as "the best time of your life." So don't waste it. Treat every day as a gift. Use nutrition to become the best version of yourself. Touch the lives of others, and always be caring and compassionate. I look forward to our journey together!

Peace, Veggies, and Rock 'n' Roll,
Alexandra

"Never doubt that a small group of thoughtful, committed individuals can change the world. Indeed, it's the only thing that ever has."

—Margaret Meade

CHAPTER 1:
Meet Your Worst Nightmare
... THE CAFETERIA

"The cafeteria deep fryer is not a toy."
—Nancy Cartwright

If you are like most students, college is the first time in your life that you are picking and choosing what foods you put in your body, how much, and when you eat. Growing up, I'm sure most of you had breakfast at the same time every morning because you had to be at school at a certain time. Similarly, your lunch was eaten at a specific time and was either packed in a lunchbox or provided by your school cafeteria. Every night you would come home and have a meal chosen and prepared by one of your parents. College changes all that. You have almost unlimited choices as to what, when, and how much you eat. For many, this can lead to eating unhealthy foods at all different times of the day, causing poor digestion and limited energy. So where does all this confusion begin? You guessed it, the cafeteria.

College cafeterias are a smorgasbord of highly processed foods loaded with sodium, sugar, and caffeine. This leads to drastic weight gain, sickness, and overall poor physical and mental health. I know it's exciting to be able to have soft serve yogurt and fries for breakfast, just because you can, but think of how you'll feel after eating that! I have also found that during my college years, I was uneducated about what was truly healthy for me. A lot of the foods I thought were healthy for me were really poisonous and toxic. For example, let's say you go to Starbucks every morning and get a bran muffin and a 16oz Frappuccino. Seems pretty healthy, right? Did you know that a sixteen-ounce Frappuccino has 6.92 teaspoons of sugar? The FDA recommends that individuals do not consume more than 10 teaspoons of sugar daily. So just in your coffee alone you've almost exceeded your limit for sugar consumption within the first few hours of your day. What about your "healthy" bran muffin? It, too, is loaded with sugar and refined grains.

Just because you don't eat cookies and candy bars doesn't mean you aren't consuming sugar. Sugar is in everything: ketchup, bread, canned vegetables, tomato sauce, peanut butter, cereal, wine, hard alcohol and most processed foods. Start reading labels and becoming aware of what is truly in the food you're consuming. Think of yourself as a Ferrari. Would you put regular gas or premium in it? The better the quality of fuel, the better the vehicle will run, and the longer it will last. It's actually very simple. If you eat crap, you will look and feel like crap.

Got the Munchies?

You've unpacked your bags, bought your schoolbooks, toured the campus, met your new roommates, and now you're hungry. The cafeteria is brightly lit with fluorescent lights and is filled with students hurriedly grabbing some grub in between classes and study sessions. The cafeteria bombards you with a variety of different foods that are highly processed, prepared in bulk, and loaded with additives like sodium, sugar, and other chemicals. In one corner are sloppy Joes, in the other grilled cheese sandwiches on white sourdough bread next to pasta with meat sauce—and let's not forget the mecca of the food court, the soft-serve ice cream station. There are so many different types of food, and so much of it available, that it becomes daunting, standing there with your empty tray, trying to decide what to eat. As a result, you pile food onto your plate and stack food on every square inch of your tray. You mix all sorts of random foods together without thinking about creating a balanced meal of greens, lean proteins, and complex carbohydrates. You slap down chicken taquitos with a slice of pizza and macaroni and cheese all in one sitting. Of course, deep down inside we all know that pizza and taquitos probably aren't a well-balanced meal, but when you're hungry and have so many options available to you, it becomes easy to overindulge.

Why do we this? In college we have the chance to exercise our newly acquired power. We are constantly trying to push the limit and experience as many things as possible. As much as we all want to stand apart as individuals and embrace our independence, we also long for acceptance and want to be the same as everyone else. When we look around the cafeteria and see our friends filling up their plates with pasta and French fries, it becomes hard not to want to eat the same things. For instance, if our new gal pal chows down on a juicy cheeseburger with warm, crispy fries, it becomes incredibly hard not to want to eat one, too. In the cafeteria our senses become overwhelmed and titillated with so many different smells, colors, and tastes that once hunger is added to the mix, it's impossible to make a reasonable decision.

In addition, food can be comforting for those dealing with homesickness and getting acquainted to a new environment. Perhaps our overindulgence can be traced back to our animal instincts. We are in a new environment with many strangers. Instinctively we may feel threatened by the flexibility of mealtimes—not knowing when we are going to get our next meal— or by the fact that the food is displayed out in the open and we have to share it with so many people. We think, *If I don't take all these tater tots now, they might all be gone if I want to have more later. I guess I should stock up on extra just in case.* This hoarding mentality can lead to overeating and result in weight gain, poor digestion, heart disease, and high cholesterol.

Put Down the Cookie!

So what do you do? For many, the cafeteria is the only place where students can conveniently get their meals. You have to eat, but in order to make cafeteria eating less hazardous to your health, you have to change your mindset about eating. Remember, humans eat to survive. The purpose of food is to fuel your body with nutrients to create optimal physical and mental performance. However, in American culture food has become more about spectacle. Eating has become an activity where food is modified into so many shapes, colors, and sizes for entertainment and visual stimulation that balanced eating becomes compromised. Do you ever find yourself eating just because it looked so appealing—even if you were unimpressed by the taste? Of course, the experience of eating colorful foods that are artistically arranged is a wonderful part of the dining experience; however, foods should not be manipulated at the cost of losing nutritional value. Fresh, organic foods are rich in color and nutrients. This satisfies your senses visually and internally. So it is totally possible to have your cake and eat it, too...well maybe not cake, but fresh vine-ripened strawberries or sweet blood oranges! Yum!

The Solution

Before entering the cafeteria or food court, take a moment to make a plan. Ask yourself questions like "Do I feel hungry?" or "How will I feel after I eat this?" Think before you eat! Once you get into the flow of your new schedule, you can find times to plan your meals and snacks throughout the day. Your body has the innate ability to adjust to your routine and will become accustomed to your new mealtime as long as it is not deprived of food for long periods of time. It is imperative not to deny your body of food for extended periods of time because it causes a dramatic drop and rise in blood sugar levels. This drastic shift can lead to weight gain and cause you to become ravenous, which usually results in binge eating or overeating. By eating small, light meals throughout the day, you will never become so hungry that you stuff your face. You will also have lots of energy because your body will not be spending all of its energy on digestion.

On a side note, it is also important not to spend all day eating, either. Every time you eat, your body has to digest your food. Digestion takes up most of your body's energy. By eating light meals throughout the day and avoiding constant grazing, you'll have an abundance of energy that your body can use to eliminate toxins, fuel your liver, rebuild collagen, and provided an abundance of other necessary functions that help keep you looking beautiful and healthy. [2]

Now back to the cafeteria. When you enter, make conscious decisions about the foods you want to avoid and remove from your diet. There is no need to go crazy and eliminate everything but lettuce. That's no way to live! Just take it step by step. Perhaps for a week or two you can just focus on trying to reduce or eliminate sugar from your diet. Then you might cut down eating red meat to only once a week. By making decisions about what you don't want in your diet, you can avert your eyes from even looking at those items in the buffet line because you've already decided you don't want them.

Also, experiment! Take note of how you feel after you eat a particular food. Do you feel sick? Do you feel bloated? Do you feel energized? Constantly check in with your body during and after the eating process. Only you can determine what foods have positive or negative effects on your body because nobody knows and understands your body better than you. This conscious method of eating can help you determine whether or not you want to keep or exclude different foods from your diet.

Now comes the fun part. Be creative. Load up on as many dark leafy green vegetables and unprocessed foods as possible. Fresh fruit is a great option, especially if you have a sweet tooth. Look for foods that are plain and are not covered in sauces or batters. The simpler the food, the more you can personalize it by adding your own seasonings, spices, or fresh herbs. One of my favorite and most convenient ways to personalize food and add extra flavor is using lemon. For example, if you have plain steamed broccoli or spinach, just add a squeeze of lemon instead of butter. It provides instant flavor without the calories and gives a zesty freshness to your food. Become friends with the salad bar. The salad bar gives you the ability to control all the ingredients that go into your meal. You don't just have to eat lettuce like a rabbit. Try adding chicken or fish to your vegetables—or tempeh, if you want a fun vegetarian option. Tempeh is fermented soy that is rich in protein and calcium and is nutty in flavor. But a word of caution: don't make the mistake of taking healthy foods and smothering them with heavy sauces and dressings. Just because you have a bowl full of fresh vegetables doesn't mean you can douse them in heavy ranch dressing. It's like putting lipstick on a pig. It might look pretty, but it's still a pig. Just because there are vegetables somewhere underneath your double cheese burrito doesn't mean you're eating a well-balanced, nutritious meal.

Bring Yo Shit, Bitch

If they don't have your favorite pomegranate dressing or that delicious cold-pressed extra virgin olive oil, find a health-food store nearby and purchase your own to bring with you. I know—at first it seems totally lame, but when you start looking great and enjoying your own personalized foods, don't be surprised if others follow your lead or ask to share! Spices are also a great low-caloric way to give your food flavor without loading up on calories, salt, and sugar. You can store them in your purse, look around and see if anyone is watching, sprinkle some on your food, and *bam!* More taste and individuality to your meal without heavy sauces or added sodium!

If you don't have a car or another form of transportation, get a group together to carpool. It can be a great way to make friends or create relationships with roommates. Shopping for food can be fun; just make sure you read the labels and look beyond the calories and carbohydrates in the items. Instead, look for things like sugar, sodium, saturated fats, and trans fats. Also read the ingredients. The most plentiful ingredient appears at the top of the list. Check labels for corn syrup, dextrose, maltose, glucose, and fructose. These items all contain sugar. Usually anything ending in "ose" should be avoided. Once you start reading, you'll be amazed by how many additives and sweeteners are found in the most unassuming foods. For instance, there's sugar in some whole-wheat breads. That's crazy! Ideal items are ones with very few ingredients and zero salt and sugar.

Swipe In!

The cafeteria can also become your own little mini mart. After dinner, head over to the fruit station and take apples, bananas, oranges, and other fruit that keep well back to your room. These are great things to snack on when you're studying later instead of that nasty box of ramen noodles. Raw, uncooked vegetables like carrots, cucumbers, or celery are also great if you can get your hands on them. Now instead of getting merely two or three meals a day from the cafeteria, you are getting snacks, too. Your parents will love that extra bang for their buck!

16

Raw fruits and vegetables are best thing you can put in your body. Ori Hofmekler, creator of The Warrior Diet states:

Living foods are the highest source of food enzymes, vitamins, minerals, and other phytonutrients in their most active state. When you ingest raw fruits and veggies, or freshly squeezed veggie and fruit juices, you reload your body with living enzymes. And every time you reload your body with living enzymes you optimize your body to detoxify and create an anti-aging effect—reduce inflammation, congestion, and pain—.[3]

So instead of loading yourself up with supplements, antiaging remedies, and diet pills, try making raw food a part of your diet. If you have the ability to get your hands on organic fruits and vegetables, that's even better because organic produce is grown without synthetic pesticides and fertilizers. In addition, organic foods have higher vitamin and mineral content because the crops are rotated frequently, keeping the soil rich in minerals. Later in the book we will discuss using the Raw Diet Movement as a cleansing program to detoxify your body of all the sugar and alcohol you've been putting in it. In my experience this is a lot easier to handle than the Master Cleanse or Lemonade Diet, and it will fill your body with nutrients and enzymes. You'll feel more alive than you ever have!

Killer Chemicals: Getting Rid of Herbicides, Pesticides, and Waxes

When taking fruit and vegetable snacks back to your room, don't forget to wash them. In a cafeteria where foods are prepared in bulk, it can be difficult to make sure that every piece of food is properly washed. While we would all hope that colleges are stocking up on USDA organic whole foods, that is most likely not the case. That means you are consuming foods filled with pesticides, chemical fertilizers, hormones, and herbicides. According to Michael Murray, ND, "in the United States more than 1.2 billion pounds of pesticides and herbicides are sprayed or added to food crops each year. That's roughly five pounds of pesticides for each man, woman, and child."[4] To avoid these serious health risks, make sure you scrub your fruits with a little soap and water. You can even purchase fruit and vegetable wash at the store to help remove chemicals and waxes. Foods that have the lowest levels of pesticides and hormones are anything with a skin you peel off, such as bananas, onions, pineapples, mangoes, avocado, corn, oranges, and so on. Again, if you have access to a car, going to the store and loading up on organic fruits and vegetables and raw nuts as healthy snacks is ideal. You can still use the fruits and vegetables from the cafeteria; just make sure you wash them.

So What the Hell Can I Eat?

Let's make it simple. We know what we can and cannot eat. We know that having French fries and burgers is probably not the best thing for our bodies—and yet we still do it. Why? For some people, it might be linked to cognitive dissonance. Cognitive dissonance is when we have to a feeling of unease as a result of two conflicting beliefs. In order to rid ourselves of this uneasy feeling, we make up justifications for the decisions we make. When it comes to eating, this can make a lot of sense. For example, you want to have a frozen yogurt, but you know that it might be better to satisfy your sweet tooth with a fresh piece of fruit. So there's your conflict. Now to reduce the dissonance, you might justify eating the soft-serve, sugary yogurt by saying, "Yogurt is a natural probiotic that helps aid in digestion, so this is really good for me." Our minds can talk us into doing all sorts of crazy things, especially when it comes to eating. Just be aware of what you're convincing yourself to do. Know that if your body is just dying to have frozen yogurt, you can have it. But then balance your diet by eating simply, cleanly, and consciously the rest of the week. Yin and yang—that's what it's about. Balance. Give yourself a little room to indulge once in a while to take the pressure off, and then go right back to your normal diet.

Now let's talk about a few guidelines when it comes to choosing foods that are right for you. Firstly, remember that it is important to keep a balanced diet. Many of us are hooked on fad diets. Some of the diets require that we completely eliminate carbs altogether, while others are composed of high carbohydrates with little to no protein or fat. Find a way to balance your diet with both. Eat lean proteins such as egg whites, chicken, fish, or tempeh. If you have the luxury of a kitchen, choose meats that are organic. Red meats should be grass fed, and fish should be wild.

When choosing carbohydrates, look for ones that are not highly refined or processed. White bread or white rice is made of the exact same grains as wheat bread or brown rice; however, the nutrients have been removed, making them nutritionally deficient. Usually if you eat white rice or white bread, you'll be hungry again in an hour later, causing you to eat more. White products have a high glycemic index, which means that they break down quickly and release glucose rapidly into your bloodstream, causing your blood sugar to rise quickly and then crash. Whole grains have a lower glycemic index, meaning that they slowly release glucose into your bloodstream, enabling your blood sugar to rise gradually while providing you with consistent energy.

When picking whole grains, there are so many different ones to try: quinoa, which is rich in protein; millet; buckwheat, which is actually gluten -free and is a relative of the vegetable rhubarb; brown rice; amaranth; barley; flaxseed; oats; rye; spelt; wheat berries; and wild rice. What's great about whole grains is that you can find ways to eat the things you enjoy without the guilt. Try having wheat flakes or oatmeal for breakfast. Go to a health-food store and find plain oatmeal without any added sugar or sodium. Throw in some fresh fruit, sprinkle flaxseed on top with a drizzle of raw honey, and you have a delicious way to start your day. Craving pizza? Make your own pizza in the cafeteria by bringing your own whole-wheat pita bread. Put a little tomato sauce on the pita, sprinkle some mozzarella or cashew cheese on top, and stick it in the oven. Voila—you have your pizza.

Be creative. Find ways to eat the things you like in a healthy way. Believe me, once you start eating organic whole foods, suddenly processed foods will no longer look appealing or taste good to you anymore.

To balance your new acceptance of carbohydrates, add in fresh fruits and vegetables and *bam!* You're eating a well-balanced meal. When choosing vegetables, dark leafy greens like spinach, kale, chard, and collard greens are best. They provide a great source of energy because they grow upward toward the sun.[5] Also incorporate some root vegetables intro your diet: beets, carrots, onions, sweet potatoes, and radishes. Root vegetables are great to help satisfy sweet cravings while providing your body with fiber.

When and Where You Eat

Timing is everything. As I mentioned before, if you find ways to plan out your meals, you can avoid being ravenous and prevent binge eating. Start your day off with breakfast. While many experts tell us to have a big breakfast, I find that you have to listen to your body and find out what works best for you. I have a light snack in the morning because I don't want to use all my energy in the beginning of my day on digestion. Think back to Thanksgiving. Aren't you usually exhausted after eating a large meal? That's because digestion takes up most of your body's energy source. If you start every day with a big breakfast, you'll be surprised how exhausted you always feel. For my personal schedule, I start my day with an organic apple, hot water with lemon, and fresh-pressed vegetable juice to give me energy and make me feel vibrant. I have a light lunch after my workout, a midafternoon snack, and then dinner. It's OK to have a slightly larger meal at dinner; just make sure you don't eat and then head straight to bed. Studies have shown that eating big meals right before bedtime can lead to weight gain, restless sleep, and poor digestion. Give yourself at least three hours to let your food digest before going to sleep.

Where you eat is also an integral part of a healthy diet and eating. I find that having lunch outside in the sunshine is a great way to enjoy fresh air and a healthy lunch. I discovered that I was less likely to rush or feel pressured to gobble down my food without the bright lights and noisy chatter around me. Outside there are things to look at and take in. I'm also not tempted to go back and get seconds because I don't see food all around me. I'm not suggesting that you become a recluse and eat alone outside, but if it's a beautiful day, tell your friends to come soak up some vitamin D!

To sum things up, moderation is the key to success. The purpose of this book is to empower you to make educated decisions about what you put in your body and decide what is right for you. Health is about balance, yin and yang—the idea of two opposite, yet complementary universes that create perfect balance. You can't have day without night or hot without cold. Too much of anything isn't good. If you eat vegetables all day long, it wouldn't be good for you because you would have an excess of fiber and alkaline in your diet. You would need to balance it with whole, unprocessed grains such as brown rice, millet, barley, or oats and lean proteins such as fish or chicken.

The same thing goes for your lifestyle. If you drink frequently, don't sleep, and have a poor diet filled with processed foods, you are going to be off balance. On the flip side, if you stay in every night and put large restrictions on yourself, you are going to feel deprived, which will cause you to binge eat or drink and go bat shit crazy. Always strive to find that perfect balance. Listen to your body. It's always trying to tell you something.

CHAPTER 2:
The Dorm: Pimp My Crib...
Zen Style

"I'm not going to vacuum until Sears makes one you can ride on."
—Roseanne Barr ."

They say that home is where the heart is. For the next few years, you'll be leaving your room at home and making a new one in your college dormitory. Not only are the rooms particularly small (and by small I mean there is barely enough room to swing a cat), but you also have to share this small space with a virtual stranger. Freshman year can be difficult for that very reason. You are constantly surrounded with new sights, smells, ideas, feelings, and most of all, people. Time to yourself can become very precious in college since you are constantly being packed into big lecture halls, dorm rooms, and party buses. While it is such an amazing experience, it is also very important to create a peaceful environment to come back to each day to help you get centered and focused. This is why your dorm room plays a pivotal role in your life. Creating a peaceful environment can be challenging, especially when living with someone else—but it's not impossible!

Firstly, when meeting your roommate, have a quick chat about your living arrangements. Ask each other questions about how you like to live. Are you the kind of person who likes to share everything, or are you more private? Do you like to do schoolwork with music on, or do you need a quieter work environment? Do you like to stay up really late and sleep all day, or do you need a more balanced sleep schedule? These are great things to talk about up front to avoid or prevent any conflict. If you both know where you stand on specific issues, you can come to an agreement and have a more relaxed and happy living environment.

Conflicts will arise during your time together. The best way to defuse tension is to talk about it right away in a calm and non-accusatory fashion. In rare cases, some roommates are so incompatible for one another that one of you may need to transfer to another living situation. There is nothing worse than dreading coming back to your room. It affects your sleep, the quality of your work, and puts a great deal of stress on you. Your room should be your sanctuary. It should be a place that is safe where you can rest, create, and reflect.

Let's talk about how to find your Zen in the college dorm. In most typical college dorm rooms, you'll find stark white walls with two desks and two beds or a bunk bed. First off, don't be afraid to move things around. Just because the room was arranged one way when you got there doesn't mean you're stuck with it. Arrange the room to be as spacious as possible. Zen living is all about space and light. Creating a sense of flow and continuity is essential to a tranquil and peaceful living space.

Once you have your room planned out, you can start filling it with your own personality. Start by organizing your things. Try to find ways to be creative with space to avoid clutter. A Zen belief is that all objects have energy. If you have a cornucopia of unnecessary objects absorbing all the energy in your room, it can be a distraction, cause you to frequently lose or misplace things, and most importantly make you feel lethargic and stressed. Keeping an open, clean space allows you to fill your room with the essentials and keeps you focused on what's important. In particular, when you add decorative pieces to your room, like pictures or flowers, they won't be lost in a sea of other useless crap. Ask yourself "Do I really need this?" or "Does this make me feel good?" Sometimes if we hold onto unimportant objects, people, or ideas, it prevents new, good things from coming into our lives. It is such a freeing experience to let go of everything. Hoarding items can be stressful and just plain creepy. Remember, less is more.

Don't Be Gross

Living in a clean space is so important in college. In college you are constantly surrounded by people and are therefore exposed to so many germs, especially when sharing a small room with another person. By taking a little extra time to throw your dirty clothes in the hamper, dust, and disinfect, you can impact your life tremendously. Try using green cleaning products. These products are biodegradable and nontoxic for the environment. If you have a little extra time and want to save some money, you can make your own cleaning products. In particular, baking soda and vinegar can be used as an all purpose cleaner just by adding warm water. Want to clean that nasty dorm room carpet? Try sprinkling a little baking soda on the carpet, and then vacuum it up. By having a clean and organized room, you will always feel relaxed and fresh. Your dorm will smell nice and no longer have that musty, stale-pizza odor. Having a clean working space is also great because it will help reduce stress. You'll never have to search through a pile of papers again to find your homework because you'll know exactly where it is. Think of all the time you'll save by never having to look for anything.

Tell Me How I'm Supposed to Breathe with No Air

College dorm rooms are often very stuffy and filled with stale air as a result of the toxic substances that fill the building. If you keep the windows open, the air in your room can freely circulate and help remove germs, giving the room a fresh smell. If you don't have a window that opens, keep the door open while you're in the room for a few hours to get circulation in the room.

Another great way to oxygenize your room is to add a few plants. Through the process of photosynthesis, plants take energy from the sun, carbon dioxide, and water and in return give off oxygen. Why is it so important to have oxygen? Oxygen is your most precious nutrient simply because you cannot survive without it. According to The Natural Health Place, "Adequate oxygen allows your body to successfully combat all microorganisms that are harmful to your body. It also allows you to detoxify chemical pollutants."[1] So trade in those tacky plastic flowers and get some real, live, beautiful plants. Some of my favorites, which are both aesthetically pleasing and provide a great source of oxygen, are Gerbera daisies, aloe vera plants (which you can use on burns or cuts), bamboo, peace lilies, mums and baby roses. Now your clean room will be filled with clean air and decorated with vibrant green plants and flowers. What a delight compared to the stale smell of beer and greasy popcorn.

Use It or Lose It!

Do you ever find that you tend to wear only half the clothes in your closet? Some of your clothes date all the way back to junior high and are so small you can barely squeeze one ass cheek into them, and yet, you still keep them. Fashion for women is constantly changing, and it is impossible to keep up. As a result, we have a variety of different trends stuffed in our closets that we are afraid to part with in the hopes that one day they will make a comeback. While I love shopping and building my wardrobe, I have a rule that helps me from holding onto things I know I'll never wear. If I haven't worn it in a year, I remove it from my closet. This helps make room for the things I love to wear and allows extra room for new clothes, a new look, and new energy.

Cleaning out your closet is fun. It feels great to have everything organized and wearable. When you finally compile enough unwanted clothes and accessories, try having a "Swap Till You Drop" party with your guy or girlfriends. I absolutely love hosting a party with organic wine and yummy treats. Have all your friends clean out their closets and bring in clothes and accessories they want to trade out. Turn your dorm room into a chic mini boutique! It's a great way to save money and hang out with friends. Donate anything leftover to charity. Now you can enjoy a clean closet while having fun at no cost.

Get Your Primp On!

Whether you're a girl or a guy, there's no denying you love to primp. Girls can spend hours making sure their makeup is perfect and their is skin soft, while guys obsess over the right amount of gel and the perfect shave. Because there are a multitude of products available that promise life-changing results, it can become overwhelming for both your body and your pocketbook. Instead of going to drugstores and buying a variety of different face washes, shampoos, and makeup, I instead suggest purchasing a few high-quality organic cosmetics.

Think about it. Your biggest organ is your skin. When you use products filled with aluminum, alcohol, formaldehydes, and sulfates, your skin absorbs these chemicals into your bloodstream. When you use natural ingredients, you will find that your skin and hair will start to clear up and have a healthy natural glow. Look for products that are 100 percent vegan, free of animal testing, free of synthetic dyes. These products can be found at health-food stores or online.

Another great way to use organic cosmetics without cleaning out your savings account is to make some of your own products. This allows you to be in complete control over what goes into your products.

Creamy Banana Face Mask:

perfect for soothing dry skin

You can get all fruit from the dining hall.

 <u>Ingredients:</u>
- 1 ripe banana
- 1 tbsp of organic honey
- 1 orange or lemon

<u>Directions:</u>
- Mash the banana up in a bowl with the honey. Then squeeze of few drops of the orange or lemon into bowl and mix. Wear the mask for twenty minutes and then rinse with warm washcloth.

Scrumptious Oatmeal Facial Cleanser:

a perfect cleanser for sensitive skin

 <u>Ingredients:</u>
- ½ cup of uncooked oatmeal
- 2 tbsp of plain yogurt

<u>Directions:</u>
- Mix oatmeal and yogurt into a bowl and gently smooth over entire face. Let sit for ten to fifteen minutes and then rise with warm water.

Sugar Plum Body Scrub:

helps remove dead skin and prevent cellulite from forming

 <u>Ingredients:</u>
- 1 tbsp of coconut oil
- 2 tbsp of raw brown sugar

Directions:

- *Mix ingredients into a bowl and apply to skin in soft circular motion for two minutes.*

These recipes are very easy to make, and most of the ingredients can be found in the cafeteria. They smell delicious and are very soothing and hydrating for the skin. There is nothing more relaxing than whipping up a refreshing organic face mask, lighting a yummy soy candle, and putting on your favorite relaxing music while you close your eyes and enjoy. Take time to nurture your body and mind. Spoil yourself! Now just add a healthy diet and exercise to your new cosmetic regime, and you'll be looking like a goddess! In addition to using organic skin products, another way to make your skin glow is to scrub your skin with a loofah or pumice stone. Many of us are good about always exfoliating our face and neck; however, our bodies get very little attention. By gently exfoliating your skin daily, you will have softer and more radiant skin and also help fight or prevent cellulite. Exfoliating increases circulation and stimulates blood flow to move fat cells.

Another way to achieve healthier skin is to end your showers with cold water. I'm not suggesting you freeze your nips off standing in ice-cold water! Just start your shower off with warm water, and then for the last minute rinse off with cold water. Cold water helps increase blood flow and provides better circulation. When you change the water temperature, your blood rushes to your organs. This helps prevent varicose veins and hardening of the arteries. Cold showers are also great because they help close pores after you've opened them up with warm water and scrubbed off dirt and dead skin. Cold water also makes your hair look shiny and healthy. That's why you have a cold button on your blow dryer. Finishing off showers with cold water will help you feel refreshed and invigorated. [2] Now you can start every day awake and energetic. So crank those showers up, and get perfect-looking skin!

CHAPTER 3:
You Are The Company You Keep

"A friend will calm you down when you are angry, but a best friend will skip beside you with a baseball bat singing someone's going to get it!"
—Unknown

In a world filled with wars, financial crises, and natural disasters, the only thing that keeps us from getting swallowed up and falling to pieces is relationships. Interpersonal relationships go beyond the mere role of boyfriend or girlfriend and include friends, families, coworkers, neighbors, and religious groups. We have a constant, burning desire to connect our minds, bodies, and souls. For example, Facebook is an entire site devoted specifically to the purpose of reaching out to people from all over the world. Within that universe, we share our thoughts, feelings, photos, and our lives. We want people to see the movies, music, and activities we are passionate about, and understand them and therefore understand us. Being with people who share the same interests, backgrounds, and beliefs as you can make you feel safe. Ideally when people come together, they use their own interdependence to influence one another by sharing their ideas, beliefs and discoveries, and therefore have a meaningful impact on the other person. Sometimes that is not the case. In some cases, our desire to be close to someone is so intense that we will sacrifice our health and happiness and overall well-being just to avoid being alone.

In college, the desire to make these connections is even stronger because for the first time we are alone. We may have come to college without knowing a single person. We are away from our families and friends and the places where we feel safe. As a result, we hold onto relationships that are detrimental to our health. College is a wonderful time to meet new people and establish a variety of different relationships with one another. For example, you might have all the same classes with a particular friend. This type of relationship consists of the time you spend together in class, doing assignments, and helping each other with the workload. Those are the boundaries of your interactions with this person, and anything outside the classroom is not a part of your relationship. You might have another friend that you drink with. She's your party friend whom you always see at fraternity events or bars. This is how we live. Certain people play different roles in our lives to give us what we need. There is nothing wrong with this concept, as long as we understand that relationships should be mutual and both parties contribute.

You CAN Talk to Strangers...Just Don't Bring Them Home

In college we are constantly thrust into different groups of new people in classes, clubs, and social events -especially when alcohol is involved. For example, you might play a round of beer pong with some cute guy who is a virtual stranger, and an hour later find yourself topless in his bunk bed…oh, college! While this example is perhaps extreme, it is very common in college to jump the gun before getting to know someone. I'm not saying you have to be a prude but in college caution always seems to take a backseat to fun. We totally forget about treating ourselves like a prize and instead give it up for a red cup filled with warm, stale Miller Light. This kind of behavior rewards people for treating you cheaply. You are worth so much more than that. Go out and do something together like grab lunch or catch a movie. Get to know each other. If you're that easy to get, people will think you're not worth having. Also, hooking up with a bunch of different girls or guys each night makes life seem mundane. Remember when you really liked someone for a long time, and then you finally kissed? Do you remember that feeling? The yummy tingles up your spine, your inability to stop smiling, the exploding feeling of joy! That's what you should be looking for. If you go around making out with every sloppy college kid, without feeling and with dead stripper eyes, you might as well charge. Establishing this type of relationship can become very problematic. Do you want to be someone's booty call? If that's how you start the relationship, it will be very hard to change those dynamics once it's been established. Why should someone take the time to get to know you and do other activities with you if you already gave them everything physically? This can be very difficult, especially when feelings are involved. As a result, you may feel stressed, depressed, and have low self-worth.

Instead, build meaningful relationships where you take the time to get to know someone. It can be such a rewarding experience when two people come together and help make each other stronger and better. I've always been a sucker for this quote: "Some people come into our lives and quickly go. Some stay for a while and leave footprints on our hearts. And we are never, ever the same." We have the power to greatly affect someone's life. We can inspire and grow and learn from one another, and yet sometimes we find ourselves doing the opposite. Create relationships with people who care about you. Be with people who make you better and push you to do things you thought unimaginable. Remember that in order to have great people in your life, you also need to be a supportive, nurturing, and thoughtful person. Treat others the way you would want to be treated. Of course for this all to be possible, you need to have a relationship with yourself and love and respect the person you are. How can someone else love and respect you if you don't love and respect yourself?

Show Yourself Some Love

I cannot stress the importance of having a healthy relationship with yourself. In a world where there is an overwhelming amount of pressure to be perfect-especially for women- it's easy to fall into self-loathing and live in a constant state of trauma. For some, this results in eating disorders, fad dieting, and plastic surgery. We are constantly surrounded with images of supermodels and celebrities, airbrushed and digitally perfected. Although we are aware of these enhancements, it still doesn't stop us from feeling inferior. We never take time to give our body the love and attention it desperately needs. This doesn't mean I'm giving you medical prescription to go on a shopping splurge. I don't believe buying material things can change your attitude about yourself. You may feel happy momentarily, but as soon as the price tags are removed, the void will reappear. You can buy all the makeup and clothes in the world, but if you don't love yourself and know your worth, you'll never be happy. The kind of love and attention I'm talking about means taking time to reflect and enjoy your own company in a thoughtful and spiritual way. Feed your body with healthy, whole, organic, fresh foods, go for a hike on a sunny day, spend your afternoon reading in the park, or take a hot bath with lavender salts and vanilla bean candles. Do something that is just for you.

Love yourself. If you don't love yourself how can anyone else? Did you ever notice that when you feel good about yourself, people become attracted to you? How can they resist? We all want to be around that positive, upbeat person who believes in themselves. We value that person's thoughts and beliefs more because they are confident and don't need approval or reassurance from anyone. This type of person tends to land the people that are most sought after because they don't need someone to tell them they are important and attractive. They already know. If someone doesn't like it, they don't care because they are too busy enjoying and improving her own life while touching the lives of others in a positive and powerful way.

"I'm going to say the one thing you aren't supposed to say. I love you…but I love me more. I've been in a relationship with myself for forty-nine years, and that's the one I need to work on."
—Sex and the City

37

It Takes Two Baby

No matter what our age or where we come from, we are all searching for the same thing…happy, healthy relationships. Ideally, two people, whether friends or lovers, come together harmoniously, creating a perfect yin and yang balance. Where one is weaker, the other is strong. Their temperaments complement each other flawlessly. They laugh, love, and live peacefully together. While these relationships are hard to find and are far from perfect, they can be attained with a little work, patience, and most importantly, communication.

Communication is everything. We can't survive without it. Both nonverbal and oral communications are used to express meaningful information between the sender and the receiver. Although as humans we possess the innate ability to talk, subsequently most of our communication is nonverbal. We communicate through our eyes, body language, gestures, clothing, and appearance. These things all say something about who we are and what we want to communicate to others.

As women, the struggle to communicate with men can be maddening. Our communication tends to be more subtext driven where there is a strong emotional undertone to our spoken words by the use of inflections, tones, and physical body language. For example, I'm sure some of us have played the ever-so-popular game called "What's wrong" to which we angrily reply, "Nothing." Why do we do this? Clearly there is something wrong, but instead of expressing our feelings we play the silent game and ignore that person's very existence. After many long and tedious hours of punishment, we finally dump our feelings onto them in an explosive and aggressive manner. For men, this is too much to handle. A more positive way to communicate is to express your feelings in a calm and collected manner. I recommend to never fight when your angry. When we're angry, all reason is lost. We are consumed by intense emotions and are unable to process the situation cognitively. As a result, we end up saying hurtful things to others and communicate by yelling and swearing in an accusatory fashion. This is not a healthy way to communicate.

I believe the best way to improve communication during altercations is to remove yourself from the situation, and take time to think and form your argument. When you are calm, then talk reasonably about your feelings and why you feel the way you do. If the other person yells, don't yell back. In Clint Eastwood's brilliant film *Million Dollar Baby*, his character says, "Sometimes the best way to deliver a punch is to step back." Instead of wasting your energy in a screaming match, get your point across in a direct and calm way. By communicating calmly, you wield more power. If the other person is not ready or able to communicate on your terms respectfully, then politely tell them you would love to chat when they are ready to talk.

Breaking Up Is Hard to Do: It's Not You... It's Me...Actually It's You!

Sometimes despite all our efforts, relationships end. While most are never perfect or easy, some relationships are extremely toxic. The yin and yang are completely off-balance causing severe stress, anxiety, and detrimental harm to our spiritual and mental well-being. These relationships are filled with tension and unhappiness, and yet we often stay in them for far too long. Why? Because we are afraid to be alone. We are afraid that no one else will come along to give us the love, confidence, and attention we need. While it may take us a long time to find those things again, we might never find them at all if we don't let go.

Have you ever been in a relationship and felt alone? You constantly hear that little voice in your gut saying, "This is not right. I need something more." Listen to that voice. You shouldn't have to rely on your friends to keep telling you your boyfriend's a douche bag or that your girlfriend's a raging bitch to get you to break up with them.

Sometimes we hold onto things in our lives, whether material objects, relationships, or jobs, because we are deeply afraid. But holding onto something prevents new and amazing opportunities from getting to you. Let go and trust that the universe will provide you with the things you need. If you love and respect yourself, you won't waste your time being with someone who doesn't let you shine as brightly. Think about all the things you want and need in a relationship, and don't accept anything less. In college, the majority of us are not married. You don't have to be stuck with one person if they are not treating you the way you want. This is the time to get to know yourself. If someone comes along and makes you feel even more incredible, than that is a person worth having in your life.

But remember, you don't *need* anyone. If you can be perfectly happy alone and satisfied with yourself, then any person who comes into your life and increases that happiness is just an added bonus. No one can define who you are or control your happiness. That is up to you. Think about it. If you surround yourself with people who care about you and make you strive to be better, aren't those the kinds of relationships that serve you best? And no matter what happens, you will always be content because you are at peace with who you are and what you want from life. Let people in, trust them, and if they end up adding stress and aggravation to your life, wish them well and gently remove them from your universe.

CHAPTER 4:
The No-Bullshit Truth
About Alcohol

"If drinking is interfering with your work, you're probably a heavy drinker. If work is interfering with your drinking, you're probably an alcoholic."
—Unknown

For many students, alcohol plays a major role in their social life. Between dorm-room parties, fraternity events, and house parties, it can become easy to drink heavily several nights a week. In the outside world, engaging in this type of behavior would label you as an alcoholic. Yet in college, binge drinking five nights out of the week becomes a common occurrence and does not raise concern because it is socially accepted in that universe. Oh, how I miss college!

For some students, this is the first time in their lives they have ever consumed alcohol or experimented with it on a regular basis. Excessive drinking in college can lead to weight gain and poor physical and mental health. What makes drinking even worse is that many times this type of behavior is accompanied by late-night binge eating of greasy, processed foods, experimenting with drugs, and making other poor decisions that can have life-changing effects. In the words of my best girl friend, "Any decision made after 2a.m. is never a good one." My intension is not to preach about how you should abstain from drinking but to provide information on the effects of long-term drinking and to dispel myths about alcohol. Then you can make decisions and find a solution that is best for you.

What Happens When You Drink

Drinking causes a disruption in the body. In Ori Hofmekler's *The Warrior Diet*, he discusses how drinking results in dehydration, depletion of vitamins, and slowing of the metabolism. The human body is made up of 75% water, and the brain is 80 % water. Drinking water helps flush out toxins and rejuvenates the cells. Hofmekler explains the importance of having a glass of water for every glass of alcohol you drink in order to maintain hydration. By abstaining from water, your cells become dehydrated and are unable to function properly. I'm sure many of you have experienced that horrible sensation of waking up with a pounding headache, nausea, and bloating. This is because you are filled with toxins and are dehydrated. Next time you plan on drinking, make sure you drink plenty of water before you go to sleep or throughout the night.[1]

Ori Hofmekler also explains that drinking leads to vitamin depletion. Through his research he found that vitamins A, C, B, calcium, zinc, and phosphorus were all depleted upon consuming alcohol. He explains that these vitamins are paramount in helping build muscle. Another discovery he made linked alcohol consumption to metabolism. This is an important one for us ladies. Our bodies naturally tend to want to be curvy and hold more fat. Hofmekler found that alcohol contains no nutritional value and is filled with empty calories. An empty calorie has no other nutrients present besides the nutrient that provides the calories. This means that you are getting zero benefits from drinking. It does not provide your body with energy, enzymes, or other beneficial components. All you get are those extra calories you don't want. Alcohol has an abundance of calories in a small volume. This means that adding a few drinks to your dinner could potentially mean that you are drinking twice the calories you are consuming through food. Your body has a set number of calories it needs to maintain your given weight. Going over the given amount results directly in weight gain.

In addition to those extra, unwanted calories, alcohol also affects the "Krebs Cycle." This is the "process behind the cellular energy production, and accounts for the oxidation of carbohydrates and fats. This cycle occurs within the mitochondria or 'power plant' of the cell, providing the energy required for the organism to function." This means that as the cellular energy begins to slow, so will your metabolism, causing weight gain and poor health. For optimal health and weight loss, we need our metabolism to burn as quickly and efficiently as possible. This requires eating small, nutritious meals every three hours, drinking plenty of water, and engaging in regular exercise. [2]

Vodka and Beer Kegs and Wine...Oh My!

I'm sure you've come up with all sorts of creative justifications for drinking your favorite beverage. For example, you might say, "Wine is good for my heart, so I should drink a whole bottle" or, "Vodka has less calories than wine" or "Beer is made from wheat, and I need lots of whole wheat in my diet." I bet you have a whole list in your back pocket to choose from. The truth about alcohol is that regardless of what you drink, it is not the best thing to put in your body. While I might recommend eliminating alcohol from your diet completely, I know in college that this would be social suicide. So let's talk about what you can drink.

I want to stress that all drinking, regardless of what you choose, should be done in moderation. I would also recommend that you never drink on an empty stomach. When you have food in your stomach before consuming alcoholic beverages, your body is able to absorb the alcohol more slowly and therefore minimize sickness. Grabbing a handful of almonds or a healthy snack before drinking may help slow the absorption of alcohol from the stomach to the small intestine and into the bloodstream.

Now let's talk calories. A single shot of liquor (1.5 ounces) ranges from 100 to 200 calories. Wine can range from 62 to 180 calories a glass depending upon sugar content. For example, if you get a terrible headache after you drink champagne (which has a low alcohol content), it is because champagne is loaded with sugar. Remember, the sweeter the drink, the more refined the sugar.

Mixed drinks are where the calories really add up, ranging from approximately 280 calories for a gin and tonic to over 800 calories for some of the more flavorful and dessert-like drinks such as a chocolate martini.

And last but not least, every fraternity boy's favorite…beer. Beer can range from 140 to 200 calories a serving. Oh, and don't be fooled by drinking light beer. While light beer has fewer calories, it still contains 100 calories or more per can.[3]

How Many Months Are You? The Birth of the Beer Belly!

Did you ever notice how many young college boys are proudly showing off their beer bellies after years of poor eating and drinking habits? As ladies, this is the last thing that we would like to happen to our beautiful bodies. How does this happen, and how can we avoid it? A study conducted by the University of Rochester explains how this process occurs. Upon consuming alcohol, the amount of fat your body burns for energy becomes greatly reduced, because a portion of the alcohol is converted into fat. The liver then converts the remaining alcohol intro acetate, which becomes released into your bloodstream and is used as a fuel source. Combine the high-caloric value of the alcohol with the storage of unburned fat, and you now have...drum roll, please...a beer belly! [4]

Lowering Caloric Intake When Partying

Of course, you want to have a few drinks with your girl friends on a night out. It would be unrealistic to think that you would completely remove alcohol from your diet, especially in a college setting. Here I will present you with a few ways to reduce the calories you intake and help keep your body looking fresh and healthy.

First, drink plenty of water in between alcoholic beverages. It is so important to replenish your body and keep yourself hydrated. Second, avoid mixed drinks like Lemon Drops, Cosmopolitans, Mud Slides, Margaritas, and so on. Mixed drinks are filled with refined sugar that will quickly raise your glycemic index (blood sugar levels) and cause you to crash later. They are also incredibly high in calories. When you have a drink, keep it simple. Have a martini with real fresh fruit. When choosing vodka, I would recommend having one that is potato or grape distilled as opposed to wheat based. Some examples of potato based vodkas are Chopin, Teton, or Blue Ice. Grape-based vodkas include Cîroc, DiVine, and Bombora. Note: these vodkas are also great if you have a gluten or wheat allergy. When ordering a vodka, have it plain and just ask the bartender to put some fresh fruit, like fresh strawberries, raspberries, or blueberries, in the shaker with the vodka, allowing the fruit to become crushed with the vodka. Ask them not to add any extra flavors or sweeteners. You just want straight vodka and the fruit.

If you're having wine, look for organic wine that has a low amount of added sulfites. Organic wines are produced using organically grown grapes. This means that there are no chemical fertilizers, pesticides, or herbicides used in the vineyard. Wines that are low in sulfites are ideal. Sulfites, or sulfur, are produced naturally after fermentation. However, some wine makers add sulfites as a preservative to prevent mold, bacteria, and oxidation. Some people have allergic reactions to sulfites and become red and irritated after consuming them.

When ordering a wine from a bar, this can be hard to track. If you are in a restaurant setting, you can pay a corkage fee and bring your own wine. Sometimes it's even a lot cheaper to bring your own, and you can control the quality of the wine and grape that you consume. Also when picking wine, lower your intake of sweet wines. The sweeter the wine, the more sugar added. If you do have a sweeter wine like Champagne, rosé, or

Riesling, only have a small amount. These wines can leave you with the worst hangovers and are filled with sugar.

In regards to drinking beer, personally I avoid drinking it at all costs. Beer tends to be very heavy in refined wheat and gluten and is usually consumed in excess. If you really do want a beer, I would try having an oatmeal stout or an organic beer made from pure grown barley and hops. Let's be real, though—what are chances of finding organic beer at a college party? And if the guys throwing the party do have organic beer, chances are they might be looking for other guys to share their organic beer with.

My last tip for lowering caloric intake is to budget how much and when you drink. If you know you are going to a party over the weekend, don't drink during the rest of the week. Also, be more rigid with your diet during the week if you know you are going to have a drink or two over the weekend. However, don't make a habit of eating really clean and then binge drinking. Be consistent. Binge drinking always leads to setbacks in your health and is very harsh on your body. Just know that if you slightly overindulge yourself one night, you can get your body's yin and yang balance back by becoming extra conscious of what you put in it before and after your day of indulgence.

And last but certainly not least, don't be a drunk mess! You know that person. The one who makes Courtney Love look like a nun. They're disheveled, constantly falling, throw up on themselves, slur, fight with strangers, become philosophical, and then cry uncontrollably. That is not sexy. People won't respect you if you're a hot mess. A sexy person has one martini and sips it slowly in between stimulating conversation. They might be a little tipsy and giggle, but they are always in control and stays cool and collected. They never make poor decisions or demean themselves because they are always in control. Now that's what I call hot.

Think before You Drink

The National Institute on Alcohol Abuse and Alcoholism defines binge drinking as "a pattern of drinking that brings a person's blood alcohol concentration (BAC) to 0.08 grams percent or above. This typically happens when men consume five or more drinks, and when women consume four or more drinks, in about two hours." Sure, drinking can be fun when you're at a party socializing, but why to do it in excess? In my college days, after a night of partying, I'd always hear my girlfriend painfully mutter, "Ugh...I'm never drinking again."

Recovering from a night out can be horrible. You wake up the next morning feeling like a truck ran over your head, your stomach is sore from vomiting all night, and you may have done or said things you regret. Remember, one night can change your whole life. Always put yourself in the position to make the best decision possible. With all these negative results, one must wonder...why do we continue to binge drink?

In college we are surrounded by strangers, and whether we want to admit it or not, we long for acceptance. We want to be liked and adored by everyone. We want to have lots of friends, and most importantly we want to have fun and experiment. Many of us won't admit that we need a few drinks to loosen up so we can feel comfortable around new people. For example, a girlfriend of mine was painfully shy around this guy she thought was cute in her anthropology class. One night at a party she saw him, but was too nervous to talk to him. So what did she do? She got shit-faced on tequila, and then she met him. Of course, by the time she did meet him, she was drunk, falling over, and slurring her words. The next day she forgot they'd even met, but he didn't. He just knew her as the sloppy, drunk mess who threw up on his shoes. Remember, you only have one chance to make a first impression. There's nothing wrong with going to a party and having a drink or two. Just become aware of what you are putting into your body, how much, and know when it's time for you to tap out and start drinking delicious, high quality H_2O.

Challenge yourself to go out one night and not drink. Can you still have fun? If you know you can go out and enjoy yourself, then you'll realize you won't have to get wasted every time you party because you'll be able to have fun no matter what. Love yourself, and know that you don't need anything to make yourself better than who you already are. If you are confident and believe in yourself, you'll wield more power, and people will want to meet you. Be yourself. Live, laugh, and have fun. This is the best time of your life, and you should remember every moment!

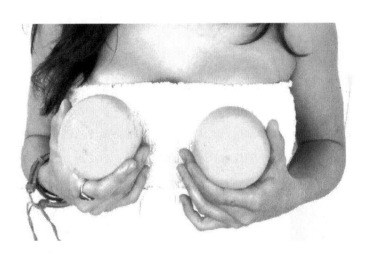

CHAPTER 5:
Oops, I Did It Again...How To Cleanse Toxins After A Night Of Shame

"Dear Tequila, we had a deal. You were supposed to make me sexier, funnier, and a better dancer. I saw the video. We need to talk." Sincerely, College Student
—Unknown

So you got a little out of hand last night. You may or may not have had one tequila shot too many and then sat down for a three-course meal of greasy nachos, a pizza snack, and a bag of buttery popcorn at 3 a.m. You're not perfect. Once in a while your emotions might get the better of you, and you will overindulge. Although you shouldn't beat yourself up about slightly falling off track, take notice of how you feel when you put nutritionally deficient foods and beverages (aka crap) in your body. The next morning you will feel bloated, achy, and your head will pound. Sometimes you'll have the spins or feel nauseous.

Think about the night before and decide if it was worth putting all those toxins into your body. Then think about a time when you woke up after you didn't overindulge. You had a martini with fresh cucumber and then drank lots of water and got plenty of sleep. It's a completely different experience. You wake up ready to start your day without feeling like you are going to die, and yet you still managed to go out and socialize without getting carried away. Well, whether you are guilty of poor eating habits or of boozing it up excessively, it's never too late to give your body the cleansing it craves to rid yourself of harmful toxins and experience more energy!

Master Cleanse = Disaster Cleanse

I can hardly count the numerous times I've heard my girl-friends proclaim that they were going to do the famous Master Cleanse, which entails drinking a horrible mixture of lemon juice, grade B maple syrup, and cayenne pepper for 10 -40 days. To make matters worse, they must also take a laxative tea daily, and the best part…no solid food.

Sounds amazing? Here's the problem. Many people experience sickness while doing this cleanse. One might argue that it's due to all the toxins coming out of your body. While that can be true for many cleanses, I would conclude that it is a result of the harsh change in diet. The other problem is that by denying your body of food, your body thinks that there is famine. Because your body's always fighting to survive, it holds on to every calorie you give it from the small amounts of nutrients it's provided. Then, when you finally end your cleanse and begin eating normally again, what does your body do? It holds onto everything you give it. Why? Because your body is genetically programed to survive. To your body, food-deprived cleanses are a form of famine, causing your body to store calories and hold weight. Once you resume your normal diet, your body may continue to store these extra calories just in case it happens again. As a result, you'll put on double the weight and will have starved yourself for nothing.

Let's look at a more natural and revitalizing way to cleanse, where you feel energetic, happy, and light without putting your body through harsh changes.

Cleansing 101

Before we talk about different ways to cleanse your body, we should first discuss what a cleanse is and why we do it. A cleanse is designed to remove toxins from the body. Some cleanses focus on the entire body, while others target specific organs. Cleanses can help promote weight loss, help with allergies, clear skin, and provide you with more energy and mental clarity. While many cleanses can cause radical changes in your diet and lifestyle, I find that cleansing in a natural way can have greater results. Cleansing doesn't mean you have to completely remove food from your diet. When cleansing you can simply choose to remove certain foods or beverages from your diet for five to ten days.

This type of cleansing is more attainable because you are not fasting and you will start to see the positive effects of removing some of these food or beverage items from your diet permanently. For example, if you eliminate dairy products during your cleanse, and then start to see how your stomach is less bloated and irritated all the time, you may decide that it might be a good idea to remove dairy from your diet entirely. Not only are you cleansing your body, but are becoming aware of how you react to certain food choices and therefore can decide what you want to eliminate from your diet.

Now let's learn about two types of cleansing I have had great success with. These cleanses can be tailored to your personal needs and goals. Listen to your body, and make conscious decisions about what you should avoid and include in your diet. You are the best judge of how you feel. I recommend keeping a log of how you feel after eliminating processed foods and beverages from your diet. Also, keep track of how you feel when you eat organic, whole foods, and try to find a way to make these foods part of your daily diet.

Spring Cleaning: Taking It Easy

I recommend starting with the Spring Cleaning Cleanse first and then moving onto the Raw Food Diet if you wish to deepen the cleansing process. The Spring Cleaning Cleanse is a gentle and easy way to begin your journey into cleansing. You know that wonderful feeling during spring-cleaning when you rid your life of all your excess possessions and make room for new, wonderful things? That's exactly what we will be doing with your body.

When doing this cleanse, don't focus on all the things you can't eat, but instead focus on all the wonderful new foods you *can* eat! Here's how it works. During a period of five days, you will slowly eliminate caffeine, alcohol, soda, refined sugar, white flour, refined grains, and red meat from your diet. Note that you can tailor this cleanse to meet your personal needs and goals. If you really want to take it slow, only eliminate a few of the items listed above, and then slowly work your way into removing all of them every time you cleanse. Also be aware that you don't have to eliminate all the items on the first day. It is a gradual elimination process so your body can ease into a new way of eating.

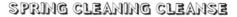

SPRING CLEANING CLEANSE

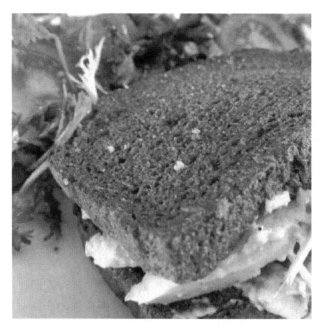

Day 1:

Remove coffee, soda, and alcohol from your diet.

For my hard-core caffeine addicts, try having green tea or fresh-pressed green juices to give your body extra energy. Start every morning with hot water and fresh lemon. This helps alkalize your body and balance pH levels. Drink lots of water throughout the day.

Day 2:

Remove all refined sugar from your diet.

Note that this does not mean you can't have natural sugar, which is found in fruits and vegetables. Natural sugars such as fructose, or "fruit sugar," and "glucose," which is found in fruit, honey, sweet corn, and root vegetables, can still remain as part of your diet. "Sucrose" is what you should avoid. It is the common table sugar found in processed foods. Try sweetening your foods with natural sweeteners such as raw honey or Stevia. Stevia is one- hundred times sweeter than white refined sugar and doesn't affect your blood sugar levels. Oh, and the best part—it has zero calories…you're welcome. And last but not least, drink lots of water.

- Add lots of dark leafy greens such as collard greens, spinach, kale, broccoli, bok choy, and chard.
- Add more whole grains such as brown rice, quinoa, whole wheat, and millet.
- Add more fruits, especially berries.
- Note: Read labels for all the processed foods you eat. You will be surprised how much sugar is found in things you would have never imagined, such as bread, pasta, peanut butter, toothpaste, tomato sauce, and so on.

Day 3:

Remove dairy from your diet.

Try having your cereal with almond milk or rice milk.

If you want to start off light, this three-day cleanse is a perfect stepping-stone to feeling great without being too aggressive with your diet. For those of you who want to deepen your cleanse, continue with days four and five.

Day 4:

Remove red meat from your diet. Stick to lean meats such as chicken, fish, or turkey. Drinks lots of water. Beans are also a great way to add protein to your diet. They are high in iron and B vitamins.

Day 5:

Eat only raw, uncooked vegetables. Start your morning off with hot water and lemon. Have fresh fruit for breakfast. Have a mixed green salad for lunch and dinner with lots of raw vegetables, sprouts, and fruit. Munch on raw almonds or seeds as a snack. Drink lots of water.

Sample Menu: College Cafeteria Style

(See Addendum #2 for added recipes.)

Breakfast

Oatmeal with fresh strawberries, raw honey, and flax seed

Find oatmeal that is unsweetened with no sodium. You can also sprinkle some flax seed over your oatmeal. Flaxseed is something I think everyone should have. It is known as one of the most powerful plant foods in the world. It can help fight the risk of heart disease, cancer, stroke, and diabetes, and is rich in essential omega-3 fatty acids, lignans, which are filled with antioxidants, and soluble and insoluble fiber. Instead of having coffee, have hot water with fresh lemon.

Lunch

Mixed green salad: fresh sliced cucumbers, mushrooms, garbanzo beans, string beans, sprouts, and a lean protein such as chicken breast, tempeh, or fish.

Use whatever raw fresh vegetables you can get your hands on. Avoid adding croutons, cheese, and heavy dressings. For dressing you can use olive oil or make your own using a little olive oil, lemon, and a sprinkle of pepper. I would avoid using balsamic vinegar. It is acid forming in the body.

Snack

Raw almonds, unsalted sunflower seeds, or pumpkin seeds
These make perfect dorm-room snacks and are also great to carry with you to munch on when you're in classes during the day. Have some peppermint tea to boost your energy.

Dinner

Lean protein such as fish or chicken with dark green vegetables
Try finding foods that are as plain as possible. Look for proteins that are not covered in sauce. You can also have mixed vegetables with brown whole-grain rice or another mixed green vegetable salad. Also, avoid eating past 8:30 p.m. because when you sleep, digestion slows and the food ends up sitting in your stomach all night. This can lead to weight gain and result in poor energy levels the next day. Have hot water and lemon.

Dessert

To help control sugar cravings, add root vegetables to your diet. Vegetables such as beets, sweet potatoes, and carrots are a great source of fiber and release sugar slowly into the bloodstream while soothing the internal organs. Next time you want cake... have a carrot. (carrot cake doesn't count.)

RAW FOOD CLEANSE

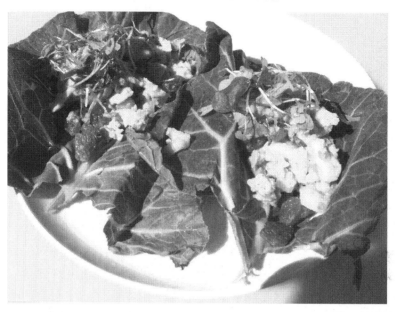

The Raw Food Cleanse is another way to deepen your cleansing after completing the Spring Cleaning Cleanse. You'll be amazed how wonderful your body will feel after removing all the sugars, refined grains, processed foods, and fatty red meats from your diet. By moving on to the Raw Food Cleanse, you will experience even more energy and vibrancy in your body.

While the Raw Food Cleanse can be a little challenging in college, it is not impossible. The central philosophy of the Raw Food Diet is to eat raw, uncooked plant foods. Food is never cooked over 116 degrees because raw foodists believe that in the cooking process, all essential enzymes are destroyed. During the Raw Food Cleanse, you will experience more energy and lightness in your body because food in its raw state is composed of living cells.

The Raw Food Cleanse can also become a permanent life-style for some people. In college this type of permanent diet can be difficult to maintain for a long period of time because it is very limited and can be expensive. You also need to have extensive knowledge about creating a balanced diet so you can get all the essential vitamins and nutrients you need to achieve optimal health through supplementation. This is why I recommend doing a short, three-day cleanse since college students lack the tools and time needed to maintain this life-style. Unlike other cleanses, you won't be starving. You'll be stocking up on lots of raw seeds, nuts, fruits, vegetables, and beans. For this cleanse, you can find some of the foods you'll need in the cafeteria; however, I would recommend going to the grocery store and loading up your little mini fridge with lots of organic fruits, vegetables, nuts, and seeds so you won't be tempted to give up on your cleanse if the cafeteria doesn't have the foods you need.

Extra goodies to pick up at the store:

- Raw organic fruits and vegetables (carrots, cucumber, dates, bananas, avocado, apples, broccoli, etc.)
- Flaxseed oil (You can take a spoonful a day or use it in a salad dressing, smoothie, or on top of your oatmeal.)
- Coconut water (filled with electrolytes)
- Raw almonds or sunflower seeds
- Raw almond butter

Sample Menu for Three-Day Raw Food Cleanse

Breakfast

Coconut water and fresh-fruit bowl: berries, bananas, pineapple, melons, citrus, apples, and figs

Try eating fruits that are seasonal to stay in harmony with nature. For example, pineapples and watermelon are great for summer to help cool the body, while apples and figs help warm the body during the fall. Have ginger tea (which aids in digestion) or hot water and lemon.

Lunch

Raw veggie salad: mixed greens and any kind of vegetables, raw nuts, or beans you want

Be creative. Eat the things you like to eat. You don't have to suffer. I love adding cucumbers, tomatoes, apples, blood oranges, mushrooms, grapes, raw walnuts, and sprouts to my salads. Think outside the box. You can add fruits and seeds to your salads to jazz things up.

Snack

Raw almonds, unsalted sunflower seeds, or pumpkin seeds with carrot sticks and celery sticks

Dinner

Raw vegetable stir-fry

Take raw, mixed vegetables such as zucchini, mushrooms, peppers, spinach, and whatever else you want, and drizzle with some olive oil, fresh pepper, and sesame seeds. *Bam!* Raw vegetable stir-fry!

This cleanse is best for those who have access to a blender. During cleansing, you can make vegetable and fruit smoothies as snack and meal replacements if you so choose. You can even make raw soups (see recipe section for details). In the dorm rooms it can be difficult to cook and prepare meals.

Although the Raw Diet Cleanse is not for everyone, I would recommend adding more raw foods into your diet. When we eat plant foods filled with chlorophyll, our blood is provided with an abundance of oxygen. Also, having a diet comprised of lots of vegetables is great if you are trying to shed some weight.[1] Vegetables are very low in calories and are filled with vitamins.

The Power Of Food: Cleansing is an On going Process

The sole purpose of eating is to nourish ourselves. Eating is not meant for entertainment; we eat to survive. Food is the fuel we need to provide us with a healthy mind, body, and spirit. Remember that whole foods have natural healing powers. For example, many studies have shown that dark leafy greens such as kale or spinach can help improve your mood and help reduce depression because they are high in the B vitamin folate, which increases serotonin in your brain. By eating raw nuts you can greatly reduce the risk of heart disease because they are rich in omega-3 fatty acids that reduce arterial inflammation. All-natural, whole foods can have powerful effects on your health. In some cases people with severe chronic illnesses have nursed themselves back to health by simply changing their diet and using food as medicine. [2]

In my own personal experience, my father had very high cholesterol that his body naturally produced. He was at very high risk for having a heart attack and has a long family history of heart disease and strokes. His doctor gave him a plethora of medications to take to help lower his cholesterol- my father disagreed. He knew there was a better and more natural way to heal his body. He didn't take the full dose of the medication, and together we changed his diet from processed foods and put him on a natural, whole-foods diet. Two months later he went back to the same doctor, and the results showed his cholesterol levels were normal. The doctor confidently proclaimed, "See, the medicine is working." My father was quick to tell him that he had not taken the medication, but instead changed his diet.

While I'm not arguing that you should stop taking medication or never see a doctor, I am suggesting that modern medicine ignores the healing powers of food and a healthy diet. In college by changing your diet you will have the energy to achieve anything you want. You will be strong, your mind will be clear, and you will be unstoppable. You will feel more vibrant and energetic and cheerful.

Chew, Chew, Chew! Your Stomach Doesn't Have Teeth!

Want to be skinny and not feel bloated all the time? Would you believe that just by chewing your food, you can completely change the way you look and feel? In today's fast-paced world we are constantly in a rush. As a result, we gulp our food down without even tasting it. When was the last time you really chewed your food and actually enjoyed the taste?

Digestion begins in the mouth. When we start eating, our mouth produces saliva, which sends a message to alert our gastrointestinal system that the digestion process has begun. The more you chew your food, the easier a time your body will have digesting it. Have you ever eaten a big meal in large gulps and felt incredibly tired after? That's because your body has to use all its energy on digestion.

By chewing your food slowly, you will also get full faster. Some studies have shown that it takes twenty minutes for our brains to recognize we are full. When we eat too quickly, we become disconnected from our bodies and don't realize we are overeating until it's too late. That's why you feel sick and sluggish. By eating small bites slowly, you will realize when you are getting full and will eat less. If you chew your food into tiny little bites, you'll never feel bloated after you eat [3] So lo and behold, you can easily shed a few extra pounds just by chewing. Add a healthy diet and exercise to that, and you'll be looking fab in no time!

CHAPTER 6:
Water...It's Not Just For Wet T-Shirt Contests

"It's clean. It's cold. Now, that's what I call high quality H2O."
—The Waterboy (1998)

With so much talk about food, one can easily forget the most important element of a healthy diet and lifestyle. Water! The human body alone is made up of approximately 75 percent water. According to Dr. F. Batmanghelidj, "Your muscles that move your body are 75 percent water; your blood that transport nutrients is 82 percent water; your lungs that provide your oxygen are 90 percent water; your brain that is the control center of your body is 76 percent water; even your bones are 25 percent water."

Needless to say, water plays a major role in achieving optimal health. However, instead of replenishing our body with purified water, we spend our day chugging coffee in between hectic schedules and endless late-night partying. By the time we finally get thirsty enough to drink water, we are already dehydrated.

Water is essential to life. Over 70 percent of the earth's surface is made up of water. Many fail to realize the power that water holds, as it helps flush out toxins from our organs, transports nutrients to our cells, promotes weight loss, aids in digestion, and provides mental and physical clarity. By adding water alone to your daily health regime, you will quickly see the positive effects that water provides you with. [1]

How Much Water Should I Drink?

You should drink half your body weight in ounces. For example, if I weigh 100 pounds, I would drink 50 0z of water a day. Your water intake can be consumed in many different ways. You can enjoy fresh herbal teas, you can get water by eating raw fruits and vegetables, and you can enjoy coconut water.

If you lead an active lifestyle or will be spending your day outdoors, your daily intake of water should be increased. Drinking plenty of pure water helps keep your skin hydrated and fresh and rids your body of toxins. When you are dehydrated you lack mental clarity and physical performance. In particular, dehydration causes your blood volume to become greatly reduced and therefore causes your oxygen supply to your muscles to decrease as well. This can make you feel sluggish and lazy.

Balancing Your pH Levels

What the hell are pH levels? Firstly, pH stands for "power of hydrogen" and refers to the degree of acidity or alkalinity on a scale that goes from zero (being very acidic) to fourteen (being alkaline), with roughly seven as a neutral point. To achieve optimal health, your body must maintain a balance of acidity or alkalinity, ideally in the middle of the scale at a neutral 7.

Different foods leave an alkaline or acidic trace in the bloodstream. People who eat the typical American diet often have high levels of acidity in their bodies. Foods that are typically acidic are meat, dairy, alcohol, baked goods, sugar, processed foods, and coffee. Having too much acidity in the body can lead to weight gain, because your body will retain fat in order to act as protection against these types of acids. To increase alkalinity levels in the body, incorporate foods such as raw, fresh fruits and vegetables, whole grains, nuts, seeds, and legumes.

Keep in mind that there is a difference between acidic foods and acid-forming foods. For example, as part of the daily routine I suggest that you have hot water and lemon every day to alkalize the body. You might think that citrus fruits such as lemon are very acidic; however, they actually have an alkalizing effect on the body. What actually determines the pH levels of food is how your body converts it during digestion. You don't have to get crazy and start reading books on pH balance. Simply make sure your diet is mostly comprised of whole fruits, vegetables and grains in order to create the perfect pH environment in your body. [2]

Coffee Is the Devil

In American culture, we are constantly in a hurry. We ignore the fact that our bodies are often completely exhausted, and instead of resting we pump ourselves full of caffeine to keep going. It is a commonly held belief that coffee wakes us up and gets us moving. While the idea of waking up in the morning and facing the world without your coffee may seem like a death sentence, it is important to know the damaging effect caffeine has on your health.

In particular, caffeine can cause a variety of different health issues such as stress, muscle tension, chronic pain, anxiety, irritability, indigestion, bowl irritation, and insomnia. Caffeine decreases the immune system and becomes a toxin in the body. Caffeine directly affects our internal organs, especially the liver, by slowing down its ability to burn fat. If you want to keep your youthful glow and a tiny waist, put down that cup of coffee!

Finally, caffeine affects blood sugar levels by causing a temporary and rapid spike. This leads to an overproduction of insulin, causing your blood sugar to crash in hours. When your blood sugar levels are constantly rising and falling, you may experience weight gain. An overproduction of insulin sends a message to your body to store the excess sugar as fat.

Speaking of fat, many coffee drinkers are not just consuming plain, black coffee but instead are loading up on sugary, dairy-filled drinks like cappuccinos, Frappuccinos, flavored lattes, and more. These drinks are loaded with empty calories and sugar. The FDA recommends that individuals should not consume more than ten teaspoons of sugar a day. In a 16oz Starbucks Frappuccino there are 8.9 teaspoons of sugar. Already in the first few hours of your day you've blown through your recommended daily intake of sugar, causing your glycemic index to quickly rise and then crash.

By starting every day off with a drug, you are setting yourself up to feel lousy for the rest of the day. Think about how you would feel if you had fresh blended spinach, kale, mangos and cucumbers (find recipes in Addendum #2). These vegetables grow toward the sun and are filled with life and vibrancy. Although caffeine may provide you with a burst of energy, your energy level will quickly crash, you'll feel jittery and anxious, and your body will become dehydrated and increase its levels of the stress hormone epinephrine (which is also known as adrenaline) by over 200 percent.

I know that giving up your morning latte may seem like torture, but once you remove caffeine from your diet, you will feel completely different. You mind will become clear, your skin will look radiant, and you won't feel bloated or agitated.[3] So pass up that cup of java and instead enjoy yummy herbal teas, zesty squeezed lemon in water, or fresh blended fruits and vegetables.

Coconut Water...A Hangover's Best Friend

There's nothing worse than waking up after a shameless night of overindulgence. Your head is throbbing, you're dizzy, your body aches, and you feel like you are slowly dying inside. While I would never recommend drinking so much that you experience this feeling, in college it does sometimes happen. When you drink, alcohol is broken down in the liver and converted into a toxic substance called acetaldehyde, which is further broken down into a substance called acetate. Acetate can cause typical hangover symptoms such as nausea and sweating. Because alcohol is a diuretic, you become dehydrated, which is another reason why you experience headaches and dry mouth.

Instead of reaching for a greasy burrito or another beer, try having some chilled coconut water. Coconut water is filled with electrolytes, which are minerals that provide the body with optimal function of muscle movement and brain and nerve transmission. Coconut water will gently replenish your body without added sweeteners or artificial flavors. These electrolytes help keep water balance in your body by maintaining water pressure within cells and the blood. This enables your body to stay hydrated.

You don't only have to be hung over to enjoy coconut water. Incorporating it in your daily diet can benefit your health and well-being tremendously. Coconut water is a good source of vitamins C and B, and provide protein, calcium, iron, manganese, magnesium, and zinc. One of the most important and essential electrolytes is potassium. Roughly 11.5 ounces of coconut water contains 680 milligrams of potassium, which surpasses the amount found in two bananas. The taste is cool and refreshing. I love having coconut water after a workout. It is wonderful for replenishing your body after a hard workout where water was lost through perspiration and breathing. Coconuts also contain high levels of lauric acid, which has antifungal and antibacterial properties that help boost your immune system and ward off infections.

Want to burn fat? Try having one or two tablespoons of coconut oil a day. Coconut oil has the innate ability to enhance metabolism because it is a rich source of MCTs (medium chain triglycerides) that help speed up the metabolism and possess antiaging properties. MCTs enhance thermogenesis, which is fat burning, have a lower calorie content than other fats and are minimally stored as fat. With healthy exercise and diet, coconut oil can provide tremendous health benefits.

You can also use coconut oil to cook with. It is great for cooking because it has the ability to remain stable at high temperatures. Coconut oil also has lower levels of polyunsaturated fat than olive oil or canola oil. While some are concerned with the saturated fats in coconut oil, these saturated fats are different from the ones found in animal products because they are short- and medium-chain triglycerides, unlike long-chain triglycerides that are found in animal products. As a result, they are processed by the body differently and are sent to the liver to be burned as energy.

You can even use coconut oil as part of your beauty regimen. Do you want healthy hair with a rich, shiny complexion? Try massaging your scalp with a little coconut oil. Coconut oil removes dandruff, lice, or helps replenish a dry scalp. It can make a great conditioner and promote growth of damaged hair because it is rich in essential proteins. You can also rub coconut oil on your skin or use it as massage oil. Your skin will be buttery, soft, and smell positively scrumptious. Coconut oil helps fight wrinkles and aging of the skin in addition to treating skin infections. This miracle oil is something every college girl should have.

Depending upon where your college is located, coconut water and oil may be hard to find. Try looking online and ordering a case. You can find great deals without having to leave your dorm.[4]

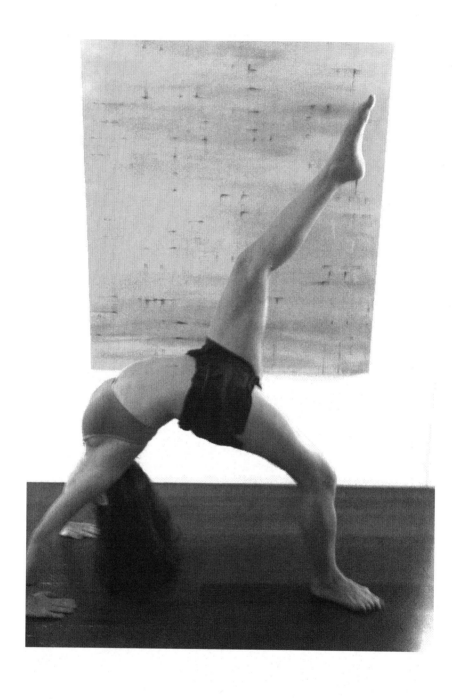

CHAPTER 7:
Time...The College Kid's Secret Weapon

"Three o'clock is always too late or too early for anything you want to do."

—Jean-Paul Sartre

In college, you can easily find yourself lost in your daily routine. In high school, you had back-to-back classes from eight to four, five days a week. Suddenly, in college, you have an abundance of extra time. You can schedule classes at times of your choosing, you can end up with large breaks in between classes, and sometimes you'll have days where you might not have class at all.

So what do you do with all this extra time? You sleep till noon, get coffee, go on Facebook, and stalk the guy you met a party the night before! Of course, college is supposed to be fun, and you are meant to have outside time to try new things and experiment. However, as you get older you'll learn how precious time is and that you may never enjoy the same luxury of time that you have in college. Most full-time jobs are five days a week from nine to six and sometimes carry on late into the night. Your weekends are filled with responsibilities such as paying bills and chores. It is so important to take the time to establish healthy eating and lifestyle habits in college because as it becomes harder to change these patterns and undo four years of damage with the limited time you have as a working adult. These habits, if carried into adulthood, can even result in illness and disease. You only have one body. It is so important to take care of it and give it the love and care it desperately needs.

Early to Bed, Early to Rise: That's Why Hot Girls Don't Have Bags under Their Eyes

Instead of staying up late every night, try going to bed earlier and waking up earlier. Going to sleep earlier and getting seven to eight hours of sleep daily is essential for optimal health. Some studies have shown that getting less sleep can increase your appetite, causing you to eat more and result in weight gain.

On average, most people need seven to ten hours of sleep to achieve optimal performance during the day. Think about it, do your friends look good after a night of partying or pulling an all-nighter on a paper they waited till the last minute to do? Usually people who do this are sporting dark circles under their eyes, have pale or gray-looking skin, are disheveled, and if drinking frequently are swollen and bloated. On the other hand, have you ever gone to bed at a reasonable hour and felt absolutely amazing in the morning? You have that extra spring in your step, your mind is alert, you're blissfully happy, and you are able to complete tasks quickly and efficiently. Creating a regular sleep schedule can improve your health and lead to a more balanced and thoughtful lifestyle. All of a sudden you can pay attention during class instead of passing out in the back row Ferris Bueller style with drool coming down your face. You'll also have something to talk about with friends besides how shitty you always feel. You'll look fresh and beautiful and attack each day with gusto because you'll have the energy to do it. Now think of adding a healthy diet to that, and you'll be unstoppable.

By getting on a more regular sleep cycle, you won't be so exhausted that you sleep till noon every morning, and suddenly you'll gain a huge chunk of free time. You can go to the gym, have time to fix yourself a wholesome breakfast, clean, have extra time to get dressed and do makeup, take care of home-work, study, or even get a jump on a paper due the following week. The possibilities are endless.

Think It...Feel It...Share It

Because of the extra time you have in college, you can really take the time to get to know your body and find out what it does or doesn't like. Make a journal and keep track of how your body responds to different foods. By taking the extra time learn about your body, you can achieve your health goals more quickly and maintain a balanced and healthy lifestyle. You can keep track of your exercise schedule, your mental and spiritual health, and your goals. For example, I might write down the foods I ate for the day and recount how I felt after eating them. Then, after reexamining the journal a month later, I might notice that every time I eat dairy, I feel really bloated so then I can remove it from my diet. Or I may notice that I feel really good when I eat lots of greens so I can add more to my diet. For my exercise, I may discover that my body is experiencing the most change when I do cardio or that my body responds well to yoga.

In life, we become so busy that our minds are not present when we experience things. We don't really taste the food we are eating because we are quickly shoveling it in our mouths. We don't think about how we feel when we eat different types of foods, we don't think about relationships we have in our lives and whether certain people are assets or are causing stress. The journal reminds us to be present. Think about things once you experience them, and use that knowledge to make your life better. You won't need to rely on people's advice all the time because you'll be able to clearly see what you need after looking back and reading your journal. (See Addendum #3 for a sample journal.)

Keep Track

One of the most beneficial books you can buy is a planner. By taking the time to write down all your commitments and deadlines for the year, you can always be thinking ahead and avoid stress. In college, one of our favorite things to do is wait till the last minute and pull an all-nighter. While you may enjoy the rush of trying to cram all your work into one night, I've found that taking your time and chipping away at an assignment can make college less stressful.

Waiting until the last minute makes you anxious and even more prone to illness. We don't always realize the detrimental effects stress can have on our lives. Some people find themselves eating more when they feel anxiety and end up stuffing their faces as a means of comfort. If you are always pushing things to the last minute and continually making yourself stressed to finish projects, you will experience distress. Distress is a negative reaction to stress, causing chest pain, weight gain, elevated blood pressure, headaches, stomach pain, and insomnia. Instead of putting your body through this experience every time you have an assignment, try planning in advance and working on it gradually before the due date. You'll have time to review your work, you won't experience stress, and you can retain more information, which is the point of writing papers and going to college in the first place.

Move It or Lose It!

Nourishing your body with healthy, whole foods is only part of creating a balanced lifestyle. Exercise also plays a vital role in your body's health and overall well-being. Exercise helps circulation, respiration, aids digestion, helps reduce stress, helps build bone density, improves sleep quality, speeds up metabolism, promotes weight loss, and provides more energy.

Today, with our busy lives and hectic schedules, exercise can easily be forgotten. You may argue that you're too tired or that working out is boring or that you just don't have the time; however, if you want to look and feel great, then it's simple: get up and get moving. In college, you have the time and the resources to get your body in shape. Now is the time to establish these habits. Upon graduating from college, you may struggle to find time to get in your daily workout. You might have to wake up extra early or make your way to the gym after working all day. To make matters harder, many office employees spend their day sedentary in front of a computer for eight hours.

In college, you have the luxury to schedule workouts as a part of your daily regime. It is so important to establish these healthy eating and exercise patterns now while you're young and have the time. Many people don't change their eating habits until they are forced to as a result of illness or dramatic weight gain. Those who establish nutritious eating and exercise practices in their youth are more likely to continue these habits into adulthood and maintain this lifestyle, even with busy work schedules and outside obligations.

Exercise...There's Something for Everyone

Getting in shape doesn't mean you have to stare at a blank wall in the gym while you're on an elliptical machine for an hour. There are so many different types of exercises for all different types of personalities and body types. I recommend always trying new things. Continually shocking and surprising your body with a variety of physical activities will help target different muscle groups and give you a finely toned body. Also, by varying your workouts, you will be less likely to get bored and stop exercising.

Working out doesn't necessarily mean you have to be in a gym. Pick things you like to do. Go hiking, bike riding, swimming, roller blading, or running outside. Connect with nature and the outdoors in places that you enjoy, like in the mountains or by the beach. You may prefer a more spiritual and strength-based training like yoga or Pilates, or maybe you love to dance.

Try taking dance classes like salsa, tap, jazz, ballet, modern, hip-hop, or Zumba. Like high-intensity workouts? Take boot camp, weight training, kickboxing, aerobics, spinning, or circuit training. My point is that there are so many enjoyable things you can do to get into shape. For those like myself who love the energy of others and need to be pushed that extra mile, taking classes is a great way to encourage you to work out. You can be in the company of others and have the guidance of the trainer to help you achieve your fitness goals.

College campuses all have gyms and classes that students can take. Don't be afraid to take advantage of this. Also, if you have extra credits for an elective, take a fitness course. That way you'll be getting your elective credits completed while working out. Taking classes at off-campus gyms or workout studios can also be fun. It's a great way to take time away from campus and put yourself in a new environment. Your workout can always be changing to meet your needs. Sometimes you may want to work out with others in a big class; other times you may want time to yourself and go for a peaceful run. Listen to your body. Exercising is not merely about physical health, but also spiritual and emotional health.

It Takes Two to Tango

If you find yourself having difficulty keeping up your motivation to exercise, I would strongly recommend finding a friend to go with. It can be incredibly helpful to have someone to hold you accountable. Together you can push one another to work hard and motivate each other to keep your workout dates. Also, working out can be a great way to socialize with friends while taking care of your body. For example, I love going yoga with my girlfriends every Saturday and then going out for a healthy brunch to catch up.

In addition to working out with friends, you can also help each other make better food choices. It's so much easier to change your diet when you have others supporting you. Keep in mind that you are there to support one another, not be competitive. Everyone's body is unique. One person might lose weight faster than another or have quicker results. It all depends on bio -individuality. See what works best for you. Listen to your body and heart and do what feels organic to you.

Kick It Up a Notch!

With twenty-four hours in a day, we get an hour's workout in at best. That still leaves us with twenty-three hours of mostly sleeping, watching television, or sitting in class or at a desk all day. The human body needs more physical activity. Here are a few ways to kick off a few extra calories and get your blood flowing.

First off, I always take the stairs. No matter how many flights, I run my little legs up those stairs. It's a great way to get your heart rate up and work your legs and butt. Another way I try to sneak in a little workout is walking everywhere. Instead of parking your car close to campus, try speed walking or biking to class. For fun you can get a pedometer to track how many miles you walk daily. Another great way to get the blood flowing is to always sit up straight in your chair. When you sit up straight, you use your abdominal muscles and strengthen your core. Combine that with some cardio workouts and abdominal work, and you'll be ready for spring break.

If you have some extra time to kill on your way to class, take the longer route. Shortcuts are great when you're in a rush, but adding some extra distance to your destination can help rack up the calories burned. Do you like multitasking? Cleaning can be a great way to burn extra calories. Put on your favorite music, work gloves, and rock out while you clean and organize your life. Dancing is strongly encouraged. By the time you're done, you'll have a sparkling clean room and get a little sweat going. Mission accomplished!

Heart Rate 101

Now that you're all fired up about working out, let's discuss the basics of heart rate. Firstly, your heart is a muscle and is essential to your survival. Physical activity helps strengthen the heart and can help can improve your muscle tone, promote weight loss, increase the amount of blood pumped to your heart, and improve your circulatory system. I recommend purchasing a heart-rate monitor to use during training. By wearing this during physical activity, you can have a better understanding of how your body is responding to the workout and train in different heart-rate zones to achieve your particular fitness goals.

Resting heart rate helps determine your basic fitness level. The better shape your body is in, the less effort and fewer beats are required for your heart to pump blood throughout your entire body. Maximum heart rate is the highest heart rate you can achieve through exercise. You can estimate your heart rate by using an age-predicted calculation. Females should subtract their age from 226, while men should subtract their age from 220.

Female: 226 – (your age) = Maximum Heart Rate
Male: 220 – (your age) = Maximum Heart Rate

When training, it is important to know that your body uses different sources for fuel depending on your heart rate. When training at lower heart rates, your body uses fat to fuel the body. When training at higher heart rates, carbohydrates are used. By training in both heart zones, you can achieve optimal health, making you stronger and leaner, with longer endurance. Spinning is a great exercise that can target both heart zones if the instructor has an equal balance of sprints and heavy climbs throughout the class. When you are sprinting on the bike, you are at your maximum heart rate. When you are doing a slow, steady climb, your body is still working hard, but your heart rate is not at its highest- it's usually around 60 to 70 percent. By constantly shocking your body with different levels of intensity, you will have a stronger heart and a more fun and interesting workout for both your body and mind.

CHAPTER 8: Time Out! Ways To Have Fun Without Being Drunk Off Your Ass

"Always do sober what you said you'd do drunk. That will teach you to keep your mouth shut."
—Ernest Hemingway

Because college life is so busy and vertically structured, we can easily forget to take a step back and look at the bigger picture. *Do I like what I'm doing or am I just forcing myself?* Be open to trying new things. They say that most college students never end up working in the field they majored in. Remember that when you're applying for majors in college, most of you are only seventeen or eighteen years old. By the time you graduate you're at least 21. The growth and change you experience in that time is tremendous. Don't be afraid to change your major or try something new. Now is the time to explore and be fearless. The whole idea of college is to provide you with a safe environment to become educated and experience as many new things as possible.

As we get older, it becomes harder and harder to change our personal and professional lives. Why? Our choices define our future path. We have financial obligations and families to support. We always keep telling ourselves that we'll eventually make a change. We think, "Once I make X amount of money, I can change and do what I really want." But we never do. One day we wake up and it's too late to pursue our real dreams.

My teacher once told me, "The man who loves his job never works a day in his life." Although every day isn't going to be a party, it is incredibly important to find something you love, believe in, and are proud of. Remember that it's not about the destination, it's about the journey.

Is There Life without Beer?

In college, spending a Friday night without a drink in your hand may seem next to impossible. Even on the nights you try to stay low key, you somehow always end up playing a "quick" game of Beirut or one round of flip cup. In college, you never want to feel like you're missing out; however, if you are drunk all the time, you will be missing out because you won't be able to remember most of it. Instead of getting toasted every weekend, why not try something new? Maybe hit a comedy club, see a play, go to a concert, go out to dinner, or check out a new art exhibit. Don't be afraid to go beyond the campus and really experience the city that surrounds your campus. Going abroad can also be an amazing experience; however, don't forget that there are so many wonderful and interesting things to explore right where you are. Go camping or hiking during the weekend, or take a road trip to a neighboring city. If your college is in Boston, try taking the train into New York. If you attend school in Los Angeles, take a drive up the coast to one of the neighboring beach towns, like Laguna Beach or Malibu.

By constantly trying new things, you'll find yourself growing and learning in a completely different way. Think how exciting life can be if you're constantly stimulated by new and interesting things. No day will ever feel the same. That's the way to live. Get out of your comfort zone, and don't be afraid to explore the unknown. By experiencing new places and things all the time, you will constantly be transforming and growing. It may even change your life. If you go see an art exhibit one weekend, you may become inspired and discover that you want to change your major to art history. This is the time to keep your eyes and hearts open. Have no judgments. Be open to new experiences before telling yourself you don't like something, unless it's some creepy drunk guy at a bar who wants to show you his van.

Don't Be a Fool...Take Classes at Other Schools!

In college it can seem ludicrous to take classes outside your major; however, now is the perfect time to try new things while you're young and have the time. Elective credits are great for this purpose. Try taking fun classes like acting, dancing, design, art, rowing, archery, singing, music, writing, film making, or editing. Do things that are outside your comfort zone—things you would never do. You might surprise yourself. It can be a very powerful thing to conquer something you are intimidated by.

During my college experience I was a terrible dancer. I forced myself to take a dance class, and even though I wasn't ready to join Twyla Tharp's dance company, by the end of the semester, I was able to do basic moves and felt more comfortable in my body. Most importantly, something that once intimidated me became a thing of the past. We are usually afraid of what we don't know. According to Titus Livius, a Roman historian, "We fear things in proportion to our ignorance of them." The more you experience and learn about something, the less you fear it. Even if you don't become a master at it, you can truly change your life by strengthening your weaknesses. You'll walk with your head a little higher and have a quiet confidence.

Even after college, I continue to take classes and explore new things. It's amazing how two completely different fields of study can help you achieve your goals. If you want to be a politician, taking an acting class can help you become a better public speaker. You'll learn to be comfortable onstage in front of an audience and begin to understand how to communicate with others to convey an idea. It's truly amazing how experiencing a variety of seemingly opposite fields of study can touch your life in so many meaningful and unique ways. In particular, I had a client who was a career counselor. I suggested he take a comedy improvisation workshop to encourage him to work with others in a group setting. What he learned from studying improvisation was that he had poor listening skills. Being a counselor, he was always used to talking and giving advice. What he was missing was actively listening to his students, instead of being consumed by his own thoughts and thinking about what he was going to say. Now he has learned to be present in the moment and allow his students to fully communicate their feelings before he is quick to provide a solution.

Remember, we are never done learning. No matter how old you are, you should always be pushing yourself to be better. During college you have this unique opportunity to take classes you want. During the summer, use that time to try more fun classes or new experiences. Try your hand at a cooking class on French cuisine, or take a class in trapeze and acrobatics. You'll be dazzled by how much you can apply these lessons to your intended career and life in general. Everything is an opportunity.

CHAPTER 9:
Brain Food: Put Things In Your Mouth That Make You Smarter...Not Sluttier

"To eat intelligently is an art."
—La Rochefoucauld

Today much of our concern surrounding food choices is heavily related to our obsession with appearance. We want to be thin, have glowing skin and hair, and look refreshed; however, it is important to remember to give the same love and attention to our internal health in addition to our external health.

If you feel beautiful on the inside, you'll look beautiful on the outside. In order to achieve optimal health, your body must be working in perfect harmony. Not only can you look great as a result of healthy eating, but you can also feel good. Did you know that food can be used to help change your moods and improve your brain function? Yes, that's right—I said it. Healthy eating can give you clarity of mind, change your moods, and increase happiness!

It is undeniable that what you eat affects not only the way you look but also the way you think and feel. Have you ever eaten a meal and then felt remorseful, angry, or just plain sluggish? Do you sometimes have trouble focusing or feel hazy? In American culture, many of us fuel our bodies with highly processed foods, sugars, and fatty animal proteins. How can we expect our bodies to perform and looks their best when we are feeding them refined, processed junk food?

Think about it. After eating sugary sweets, you'll experience a rush of energy that lifts your mood and spirit, but quickly after comes the sugar crash making you feel tired, aggressive, or depressed. Although eating is an enjoyable activity, food is not meant for entertainment, but rather a means to nourish your body and provide you with energy. The more high-quality foods you feed your body, the better your daily performance and overall health will be.

Your body loves you. Love your body back. It wants to survive and will run as best it can on what you give it. By giving your body whole, fresh foods, you will receive life-changing benefits.

Put Down the Lexapro...Pick Up a Carrot

Don't you wish there was a pill you could take that would replace exercise and a sensible diet? In today's day and age, we are always quick to solve our problems with a pill, having little knowledge about what we are putting into our bodies and unwilling to find ways to prevent our health problems entirely. In college, we are bombarded with tests, papers, classes, projects, and social events. It is a time where we are expected to challenge ourselves and push beyond our limits. Yet since we are in an environment lacking the constant support of our family and closest friends, we can easily feel stressed and anxious.

To make matters worse, the food being provided to college students is usually poor quality and highly processed. Now is the time to be very aware about what you are putting into your body and how it makes you feel. The types of foods you choose and the way in which they are prepared, combined, and consumed all have an effect on the way you feel, changing your mood and energy levels throughout the day. I never would have imagined that I could pull myself out of a bad mood or slump by simply changing the way I ate. It is a truly magical feeling to have more control over your emotions while having more energy and zest throughout the day. So, let's talk about our brains.

Our brains communicate by chemical substances called neurotransmitters. Neurotransmitters have the ability to affect mood, temperature, sleep, appetite, and heart rate along with many other functions in the body. According to modern science, the foods we eat have the ability to cause changes in these neurotransmitters. The neurotransmitters that are most affected by diet and have a strong connection to mood are serotonin and dopamine. Serotonin is known to be a calming and relaxing chemical in the body. Studies have shown that when we eat carbohydrates, serotonin is released into the body and has a calming and soothing effect. However, let's remember that all carbohydrates are not created equal. Carbohydrates are classified into two groups: simple and complex. While both groups of carbohydrates contain sugar, they are processed by the body differently and can have positive or negative effects depending upon the type carbohydrate.[1]

93

Simple and Complex Carbohydrates

Simple carbohydrates are typically highly processed and contain refined sugars. Examples of simple carbohydrates are processed foods like bagels, cookies, sugary cereals, and pastas. The rule of thumb for simple carbohydrates is to avoid white foods. If it's white, it ain't right. Think of how fluffy and light Wonder Bread is. That is because all the essential vitamins and minerals have been removed from the grain. Now think of pure whole-wheat bread. It is dense, with a darker, rich brown color. These two different types of carbohydrates will provide you with different energy levels. This is linked directly to blood sugar levels and sugar intake.

Pour Some Sugar On Me

Because refined sugars, called sucrose, are used in processed simple carbohydrates, they cause our blood sugar to rise rapidly. Have you ever eaten a lot of sweets on Halloween when you were a kid and gotten a sugar high? You had a sudden burst of energy and then completely crashed an hour later. Refined sugars quickly enter the bloodstream after they are eaten. Your body then goes into an emergency state because of the high sugar levels present and attempts to burn the energy quickly, hence the sugar rush followed by the crash once the energy is quickly burned.

Now, I don't want you to think all sugar is bad. Truth is…it's not. Only white, refined sugars are the culprits of weight gain and premature aging. Naturally occurring simple sugars found in fruit, called fructose, when eaten in moderation, are fine as a part of your diet. For example, the sugar found naturally in fresh fruit does not cause a rapid sugar rush because fruits are also rich in fiber. The fiber slows the rate at which the sugar is being digested, causing a slow and steady rise. When sugar is digested, it becomes glucose in the body; glucose helps provide energy to your body's cells.

Depending upon the type of sugar you eat, sugar enters your bloodstream and becomes converted to glucose at different rates. The measurement of the rate at which sugars from different foods are converted to glucose is called the glycemic index (GI). Keep in mind that just because some foods have a high GI, like carrots or bananas, doesn't mean they should be removed from your diet. Fiber from carbohydrate sources like vegetables, whole grains, and fruits actually helps stabilize blood sugar levels.

Now that we understand sugar levels in carbohydrates, let's talk about good carbs. These are called complex carbohydrates. Unrefined complex carbohydrates are a great source of energy. Complex carbohydrates include fresh fruits, vegetables, and whole grains. Attempting to find pure whole grains can be difficult. When strolling down the aisles of your local grocery store, you'll see the words "whole grains" splashed across every box. However, most of these items contain minuscule amounts of whole grains, if any at all. When choosing your whole grains, look at the ingredients of the product. Look for ingredients such as whole wheat, brown rice, oats, and rye. Avoid ingredients like cornstarch, white enriched flour, added coloring, and preservatives. Also, look at the sugar content. You'll be amazed how much sugar you'll find in whole-wheat bread or white flour pasta.

When I choose my whole grains, I usually avoid processed foods and choose something I make myself. There are an abundance of pure whole grains to choose from that are rich in vitamins and minerals such as quinoa, millet, rice, amaranth, barley, buckwheat, corn, flax, kamut, oats, and spelt. These carbohydrates have long chains of sugar that are bound with fiber. When digesting these foods, your body breaks down the chains of sugar and releases the fiber into your bloodstream. As a result, you'll be provided with a consistent amount of energy because it has a low glycemic index that raises your blood sugar gradually. Starting your day off with rolled oats is perfect for keeping your energy up throughout the day, and it helps reduce hunger cravings.

Now that we understand complex carbohydrates, lets discuss other foods that have a strong connection to your energy levels and feelings. The other neurotransmitter that has a strong connection to mood is dopamine. Dopamine has been shown to have an energizing effect on the body. Meals that help produce dopamine contain lean protein and are low in fat. Diets that include a combination of complex carbohydrates, lean proteins such as (e.g. fish, nuts, and sprouts) and fiber (whole, organic fruits and vegetables) are perfect for providing your body with enough energy to attack your day.

Healing Your Brain One Tasty Nut at a Time!

Yes, I said it. Fill your mouth with nuts! Walnuts have been around for millions of years and have been deemed by historians as a prehistoric food used by hunter-gatherers. In recent studies, walnuts have been called "brain food." In particular, walnuts are rich in nutrients and are filled with minerals, vitamin E, and antioxidants. Unlike other nuts, walnuts contain omega-3 fatty acids and alpha-linoleic acid. Omega-3s are an essential fatty acid that your body does not produce naturally and can only be acquired through diet. Omega-3s play a vital role in healthy brain and nerve function. If you're not a big fan of fish, or if you're a vegetarian, walnuts will efficiently provide you with omega 3s needed to maintain a healthy and balanced diet.[2] Walnuts are also rich in protein and fiber and help lower cholesterol.

Nuts and seeds can make great snacks or toppings on salads or desserts. Keep your nuts in a sealed container in the refrigerator to keep them fresh. I also recommend soaking nuts and seeds before eating them to rinse off natural inhibitor enzymes. This will make the nutrients more readily available. When you don't soak nuts and seeds, they can be more acid forming in the body. Soak nuts overnight in one or two inches of water until they are plump from absorbing all the water. You can then gently rinse them off and start enjoying them.

Some of my favorite nuts and seeds to snack on are pecans, walnuts, almonds, hemp seeds, chia seeds, sunflower seeds, sesame seeds, coconuts, and pine nuts. Because nuts are a calorically dense food, I recommend enjoying them in small portions daily. Nuts and seeds are an excellent source of protein and should always be eaten raw. A handful of raw nuts are a much healthier late-night snack than a bag of chips or a slice of pizza. Nuts and seeds also make great snacks to keep in your purse to munch on in between classes, when you have to go longer periods between meals, or when you have back-to-back classes.

The Brain Grain

Quinoa, known as a super grain, is highly nutritious and can supply you with all of the body's requirements: carbohydrates, fats, protein, vitamins, minerals, and fiber. While most grains are deficient in the amino acid lysine, quinoa has an adequate quantity of lysine and contains all the essential amino acids, making it a complete protein. Quinoa is said to have the ability to help improve memory. It is rich in folic acid, zinc, vitamin E, and iron. Quinoa is gluten- free and considered an ideal food for those prone to food allergies.

Quinoa is so easy to cook and can be paired with anything. I love adding quinoa to my salads. Because it is a complex carbohydrate, it will fuel you with consistent energy and get you through a long day of studying.[3]

An Apple a Day Keeps the Doctor Away... and Keeps You from Losing Your Marbles

When in season, apples make a wonderful snack not just because they are tasty but also because they help fend off degenerative diseases like Alzheimer's. This is because the skin of apples is rich in antioxidants, minerals, and most importantly a nutrient called quercetin. Quercetin is even more powerful than vitamin C when it comes to fending off disease. It is classified as one of the many flavonoids that give plants their color and are potent antioxidants that help neutralize free radicals in the body. Next time you're running to class and need a snack along the way, throw an apple in your bag![4]

Onions...Peel Away Toxins One Layer at a Time!

Although they can be potent, try incorporating raw onions in your diet. I love adding them to salads with fresh greens or to my homemade guacamole. Once you cook onions, the natural enzymes with amazing healing properties are destroyed. Like apples, onions contain flavonoids, in particular a flavonoid called fisetin that is found in fruits and vegetables. Studies have shown that fisetin helps improve memory by alerting pathways that boost long-term memory. In addition, onions are also wonderful for building connective tissue in the skin, such as collagen. Also, because onions are rich in sulfur, they help clean the liver, which is our main fat-burning organ. The liver uses bile to push excessive fat out of the body and into the small intestines. A diet rich in fiber from fruits, veggies, and whole grains causes the unwanted fat to be released from the body every time you hit the bathroom. Next time you want to binge drink after playing two rounds of beer pong, think of your liver! Swelling and inflammation may occur in the liver after heavy drinking for an extended period of time. How are you supposed to shed that extra fat when your liver is suffering after a night of boozing? Be good to your liver...it wants to be good to you![5]

Stop Texting on Your Blackberry and Pick Up Some Blueberries!

Berries are truly a beautiful superfood. They are rich in antioxidants and protect the brain against memory loss. Blueberries are the best source of antioxidants; in a study conducted at Tufts University, sixty fruits and vegetables were analyzed for antioxidant potential, and blueberries were ranked as the highest. Like apples and onions, they are rich in flavonoids that give them their rich blue, purple, and red pigments. Blueberries are rich in vitamin C and fiber, both soluble and insoluble. The antioxidants in blueberries provide the brain with protection from oxidative stress and combat age-related conditions such as Alzheimer's. Further studies have shown that including blueberries in your diet daily dramatically improves motor skills and the ability to intake information. Blueberries are also rich in water and fiber and help regulate your blood sugar while alleviating sugar cravings. Best of all, these berries are rich in phytonutrients, which are organic components of plants that promote health and wellness by collaborating with vitamins and minerals in the body.[6]

Incorporating these superfoods into your diet is incredibly easy and inexpensive and can have life-changing effects on your physical and mental health. I like to add a cup of fresh blueberries to my oatmeal every morning or to fresh fruit smoothies. I encourage you to buy organic, if possible, to avoid pesticides and synthetic fertilizers. Look for berries that are firm and rich in color, and make sure to wash them thoroughly just before you eat.

I also suggest eating seasonally. For example, apples are naturally ripe in the fall. We eat certain foods at certain times of the year because they provide our bodies with unique properties that help cool or warm us depending upon the climate. For example, in the summer we enjoy cooling fruits and vegetables like watermelon, cucumbers, and pineapples because they help hydrate the body and keep us cool when it's hot outside.

Likewise, in the fall when it becomes chilly, we enjoy chestnuts, figs, squash, and pumpkin to help warm the body. When you eat seasonally, you can begin to enjoy seasons and feel a strong connection to the earth. Also, the foods you eat will be ripe and delicious. What better way to look sensational and stay grounded?

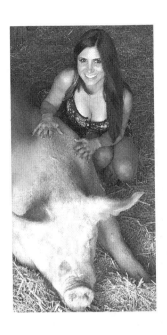

CHAPTER 10:
The Conscious College
Student

"I love mankind, it's people I can't stand."
—Peanuts

In college, we are impulsive. We do things without thinking about the effects they have on others and ourselves. We eat too much, drink too much, and do everything in excess. While college is the perfect opportunity to experiment and test our limits, we sometimes forget that if we approach things cognitively, we can make better choices and use our newfound freedom to create change and impact other people's lives.

One thing the average college student is guilty of is being wasteful. According to Dump and Run, a nonprofit that provides waste prevention education to college campuses, "the average college student produces 640 pounds of solid waste each year, including 500 disposable cups and 320 pounds of paper." Similarly, a study conducted at Tufts University showed an astounding increase in the university's waste production every spring when students prepare to leave campus. For example, in 1993 the university produced 50 tons more waste than the average 180 tons that is produced yearly.[1]

What's unique about college, unlike any other community, is that despite the diverse cultural, religious, and economic backgrounds, everyone is facing the same challenges and experiences. We are all trying to find ourselves. We want to know who we are and what we stand for. College brings together a group of young individuals hungry for knowledge and new experiences. If you can combine forces with your peers and school administration, you'll be amazed by all power you have. College students often are unaware of the power they hold. Right outside your dorm room you have access to a plethora of like-minded and eager individuals who are anxious to use their newly acquired freedom.

Gorgeously Green

Be the catalyst for change on your college campus. If you want to promote a more eco-friendly college environment, start a petition. You can approach the school administration and create a proposal to add recycling bins in dorms and throughout the campus. However, recycling is just the beginning. There is a multitude of ways to make your campus green, and it all starts with you. Campuses can change the way they maintain school grounds by using food waste as compost to fertilize flowers and grass. They can use hybrid cars for student shuttles or staff members to use on campus. They can use solar energy panels to power buildings. Assignments and course handouts can be posted online instead of printed, teachers can use double-sided printing for tests to cut down on wasted paper, and administrators can install low-flow shower heads and faucets in student-housing facilities.

There are so many ways to be creative and work together to build a gorgeously green campus. Not only will the students and faculty benefit from your program, but the university will prosper as well. According to The National Recycling Coalition,

> Well-designed programs save money. Communities have many options available to make their programs more cost-effective, including maximizing their recycling rates, implementing pay-as-you-throw programs, and including incentives in waste management contracts that encourage disposal companies to recycle more and dispose of less.

A recycling program costs less to run and operate than waste collection. The more people recycle, the more costs become inexpensive. Ideally, the university could use this newly acquired income to make improvements on campus or support local student groups.

While I know that starting rallies and petitions might be a big first step for you, you can also make small changes in your daily life that can have a tremendous effect.

Making your room a chic, eco-friendly environment can be incredibly easy and economical. Being healthy is not only about making you look gorgeous on the outside, but also about feeling good on the inside. Being a part of something bigger than yourself is truly an astonishing experience. It makes you realize that no matter what happens at the end of each day, you contributed in some small but powerful way. Here a few easy steps to make your dorm fabulously green.

Recycle (Books, Not Boys)

If the dorm does not provide a recycling bin, set up one in your room. Not only can you recycle plastic, but you can also recycle paper, electronics, and ink cartridges—and you can even make a little extra cash doing it! Some companies are willing to buy used ink cartridges or cell phones. Now you can help the environment while picking up a few extra dollars. That's what I call a win-win.

Another way to recycle is to buy used books online or on campus. At the end of the semester, instead of burning your English lit books, pass them along by either selling them back to the bookstore, selling them online, or giving them to charity...cause misery loves company.

Quick Fixes: Less Is More

Next time you decide to sing the entire Britney Spears ... *Baby One More Time* album in the shower, save it for karaoke.

Taking shorter showers is a great way to save water. By keeping showers to ten minutes or less, you can save thousands of gallons of precious H_2O. Then you can be clean and green!

Another easy trick to take your dorm from drab to fab is to remove those artificial crappy air fresheners and instead use fresh live plants. Indoor plants can improve air quality and give your room a tranquil and inviting ambience. I love white orchids because they are beautiful and easy to maintain.

Another easy way to spruce up your dorm is to use compact fluorescent light bulbs instead of those nasty overhead dorm-room lights. Decorate your room with a few lamps, or use natural lighting when possible.

Is it getting hot up in this bitch…? Lose the air-conditioning and turn on a fan or open a window. Fresh air has the power to provide you with a steady supply of oxygen that is essential for optimal brain and cell function. By staying in a confined, closed area for extended periods of time, such as the dorm room, library, or classroom, you will be breathing in the same stagnant air over and over again. Over time the oxygen content in the room will diminish because we breathe in oxygen and exhale carbon dioxide and other toxins. In contrast, fresh air is rich in negative ions that are filled with oxygen. In particular, oxygen possesses a negative charge, while carbon dioxide carries a positive charge. The higher the oxygen content, the more negatively charged the room will be. So get rid of that nasty, stale air, and open a window!

Unplugged

An easy way to save on energy is to unplug any electronics you are not using. Also on a health note, it is imperative to reduce your exposure to electromagnetic fields (EMFs), which have been found to be cancer-causing agents. You can do this by reducing cell phone use and by keeping electrical devices away from your bed. If you use alarm clocks or radios near your bed, make sure they are battery operated. Similarly, you can save energy and lower your monthly electricity bill by turning off lights when you are not using them.

You Can't Facebook If You're Using a Notepad

Next time you head to class, leave behind your notebook and bring a small laptop. You can save tons of paper by writing all your class notes on your computer. It can also help you be more organized and efficient. Now you can easily organize all your class notes in one compact unit. You'll have more space and use fewer materials. When you walk to class, your tote bag won't be stuffed with six binders and notebooks, but instead you'll have one light computer and a folder with handouts and homework.

Another perk about taking notes via computer is that it is much faster to type and take notes than to write. You'll never have to be that kid on the first day of class asking, "Does anyone have a pen?" Your life will be more convenient and eco-friendly. Besides, now you have a great excuse for making your parents buy you that cute mini laptop you've been wanting.

Be Smug with Your Mug!

Next time you sashay your sexy little booty into the campus coffee shop to get a quick pre-class coffee or tea, bring your own mug. Disposable cups are so nineties! It's time to add a little personal touch to your beverage experience. Why not sport a cute thermos to drink your vanilla spice tea, decorated with fun pictures of you and your friends? Hell, you can even drink out of a pimp cup, as long as you are saving the environment from excess disposable waste. That's right...I said it. Save the environment one pimp cup at a time!

Killing the Environment—One Toga Party at a Time!

Speaking of pimp cups, this brings me to my next point. Have you ever been to a house or frat party and seen a sea of red cups? In the morning these cups encompass the entire floor, some dripping with stale beer, others are filled with cigarette butts. While it is clear there was a rager the night before, what isn't clear is where all these shiny fire engine red cups go. In the best of situations, you might hope these cups make their way into the blue recycling bins; however, even these cups still find their way into the landfills. Here's why. Have you ever looked at the bottom of your plastics and seen a number? These numbers are "Plastic Identification Codes," which correlate to how difficult or easy something is to recycle and what type of packaging it has. Number 1 is the easiest, and number 7 is the hardest. Where you live also determines what types of plastics you can recycle because different communities handle recycling differently. Red cups are typically rated as a number 6. They are made out of polystyrene and are considered a single-use item. Polystyrene is the most difficult plastic to recycle for two reasons: it is more expensive to recycle than to create from raw materials, and it is often contaminated by food or beverages.[2]

So how do you fix this problem? It's simple. If you're hosting a party, use cases of beer instead of getting a keg. These cans and bottles are much easier to recycle. Another way to change things up is to stop purchasing red cups. I know they are an icon of the epic college party, but let's face it...beer is beer no matter what cup it's in. Look for plastics that have numbers 1, 2, or 7. Make sure the plastic does not say 6PS; these cannot be recycled. Or why not be classy and rock a flask?

While I am not advocating drinking, I can't argue that it is not a part of college life and doesn't happen. While for many health reasons I encourage you to limit drinking and be picky about what you drink, it's also important to become aware of eco-friendly ways to throw parties without killing our beautiful environment.[3]

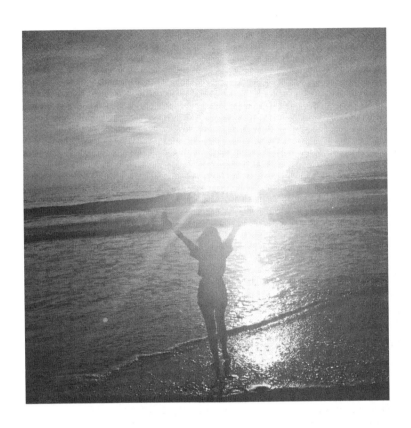

Conclusion

"You're on your own. And you know what you know. And you are the one who'll decide where to go…"
—Dr. Seuss

N ow that you have learned to create a balanced and nutritious lifestyle for yourself and the environment, it's up to you to discover what you want your college experience to be. Experiment, try new things, but always be kind to yourself. You only get one body. Nurture it. Make a goal to do something fun every day that is just for you—basking in the sun, reading a good book, taking a brisk walk, cooking yourself a delicious meal, meditating, praying, or simply taking time to reflect and send yourself some love.

What are you grateful for? We often spend a lifetime obsessing over all the things we want. But how often do we sit and relish all the wonderful things we have? Take time to work toward larger goals, but remember that you already have so much. Every day is a gift. Even when everything falls to pieces before your eyes, there is always something to be learned or gained.

And most importantly, remember to enjoy college. Life can get crazy with term papers and parties and friends and tests. Take the time to stop and enjoy it. You'll be amazed at how quickly four years goes by. This is the best time of your life. Take the time to get to know yourself and love who you are. Start each day with an open mind and an open heart, without fear or judgment.

If you take one thing away from this book, this is what I want you to keep in your heart: life is a journey. You are never going to stop growing and learning and discovering who you are. There is no rush. Never make decisions based on fear. Do what feels natural and organic to you. It's not about the destination…it's all about the journey.

With love, light, and laughter,

Alexandra

"Life moves pretty fast. If you don't stop and look around once in a while, you could miss it."
—Ferris Bueller

Addendum #1: Shopping List

Here is a list of some items you might want to stock in your refrigerator. You do not have to buy all these products. This list is to help guide you to foods you might want to include in your diet. While purchasing organic vegetables is always best, if you do purchase nonorganic produce, make sure to wash it thoroughly to remove chemicals and pesticides. Most importantly, eat what you like. Choose foods that are both nourishing for your body and your taste buds!

Fruits

- Apples
- Bananas
- Berries (blueberries, blackberries, raspberries, strawberries, goji berries)
- Citrus (lemons, limes, oranges, nectarines)
- Cherries
- Coconut

- Figs
- Grapes (don't buy seedless; that means the food has been genetically modified)
- Grapefruit
- Mangos
- Papaya
- Pears
- Pineapple
- Pomegranates
- Plums
- Watermelon

Vegetables
- Arugula
- Asparagus
- Avocado
- Broccoli
- Carrots
- Celery
- Corn
- Cucumber
- Green beans
- Kale
- Mushrooms
- Onions
- Radishes
- Romaine lettuce
- Snap peas
- Spinach
- Sprouts (alfalfa, bean, or green leaf)

- Tomatoes

Oils

- Coconut oil (organically grown and unrefined)
- Cold-pressed extra-virgin olive oil
- Grape seed oil
- Raw, unrefined apple cider vinegar

Grains

- Brown rice
- Buckwheat
- Kamut
- Millet
- Quinoa
- Whole wheat (Ezekiel Bread)

Spices:

- Black pepper
- Basil
- Cayenne pepper
- Cinnamon
- Curry Powder
- Oregano
- Turmeric

Nuts and Seeds

- Almonds
- Chia Seeds
- Flaxseed
- Hemp seeds
- Pecans
- Pine nuts

- Pumpkin seeds
- Sunflower seeds
- Walnuts
- Young Thai coconuts

Sweeteners

- Raw cacao
- Raw honey
- Stevia
- Vanilla extract

Milks

- Almond milk
- Coconut milk
- Hemp milk
- Rice milk

Condiments

- Celtic or Himalayan sea salt
- Dijon mustard
- Tamari
- Tahini

Spirit and Spice...and Everything Nice

Celtic or Himalayan Sea Salt

Unlike bleached salt, from which all the nutritional value has been removed, sea salt is rich in minerals and trace elements such as magnesium, chloride, and potassium. Another perk of sea salt is that it does not contribute to high blood pressure. Adding a little harvested sea salt in moderation will add flavor to your meals while providing a plethora of essential enzymes, elements, and minerals.

Raw Honey

Raw honey is great when used in moderation as a sweetener. It is a whole, natural food that is enzymatically active and is rich in iron, manganese, B6, and riboflavin. Raw honey contains live bacterial cultures that help promote digestion and absorption of nutrients. Unlike your favorite "honey bear," raw honey has not been pasteurized, which means it retains all the phytochemicals that are destroyed during the heating process. Darker honey contains flavonoids that provide the body with antioxidants. Next time you want to sweeten your tea with sugar, instead reach for some raw honey.

Miso

Miso is a great addition to salad dressings or if you have a stove, to make soup. Miso is a fermented soybean paste that is rich in minerals such as phosphorous, zinc, manganese, iron, and copper. Miso helps boost your immune system, is a natural probiotic (which helps put good bacteria back into your body), and is high in protein and potassium. I love adding miso to my salad dressings to help make them creamy and rich without using milk or cheese. Look for unpasteurized miso. I also suggest getting light miso because it's not as salty and has a subtler flavor. You can typically find miso at Whole Foods or local health markets.

Cayenne Pepper

Cayenne pepper is great for spicing up veggie dishes and teas while providing you with a multitude of health benefits. In regions throughout the world such as Mexico, Southeast Asia, and China, cayenne pepper has been used as medicine to treat an extensive array of ailments such as sore throats, digestive issues, fever, infections, and asthma; it also is used to improve digestion. Cayenne pepper is rich vitamins such as carotene and vitamin C. Remember, a little sprinkle goes a long way. It will last you forever!

Addendum #2: Easy and Delicious Recipes

In college, most of us don't have the luxury of a kitchen with an oven and stove readily available. Most dorm rooms just have a small refrigerator and microwave. The following recipes I have created are simple and can be made in any college dorm room. Now you won't have to spend all your parents' money on crappy vending machine snacks or cafeteria food. So throw out those ramen noodles and stock up on fresh veggies and fruits.

Bad-Ass Power Tools

1. Blender

   Because you probably don't have access to an oven or stovetop, most of the recipes below are raw. I try to avoid using the microwave as much as possible because it can be harmful to your health. Unlike ovens, microwaves are composed of high-frequency waves of electromagnetic energy that force the molecules in your food to move incredibly fast to create heat. Microwaves are so powerful that the radio waves can pass through glass and plastic. One of the major concerns with microwaves is they produce a particular type of radiation called non-ionizing radiation. Although non-ionizing radiation is not as toxic as ionizing radiation (which has the ability to change your DNA), it is still radiation nevertheless. All you have to do is be careful around your microwave and don't stand directly in front of it just in case of radiation leakage.

This is why for the most part I use a blender, and create tasty raw treats instead of cooked ones. I recommend spending a little extra money and getting a good-quality blender. You'll be surprised how many meals you can make with a blender, from smoothies to salad dressings, soups, desserts, sauces, and more.

2. Cutting board
3. One kick-ass sharp knife
4. Mixing bowls
5. Plastic containers to store food

Note: These recipes were created to be simple and easy so that these foods can be made in a dorm room or cafeteria without the use of an oven or stove. Feel free to use them merely as a stepping-stone to creating your own healthy meals. Whatever satisfies you and leaves you feeling energized and vibrant is what you should be eating.

Breakfast: Fruits, Veggies, and Whole Grains

While we would all love to have the time to make a nutritional breakfast every morning, in college it can be difficult. Below are some quick suggestions for healthier options to foods you might normally enjoy.

- If you use instant oatmeal, look for gluten-free oats that do not contain any sodium or sugar.
- Switch up your milk for almond or rice milk.
- Have fresh fruit instead of pastries in the morning.
- Instead of coffee, try some hot water and lemon or fresh herbal teas.
- Switch from eggs to egg whites.
- Instead of using sugars to sweeten foods and beverages, opt for raw honey and cinnamon.
- Instead of a bagel with cream cheese, have whole-wheat toast with fresh crushed strawberries and honey on top, or a drizzle of almond butter.

Just a few simple switches in your food choices can be a great way to help shed extra pounds while still enjoying your favorite breakfast treats. Eating lighter during the morning and afternoon is ideal. When you have a heavy, large breakfast, all your energy will go toward digestion, leaving you feeling tired as you start your day. Starting your day off light and moving to heavier foods toward the early evening is ideal. You'll feel more energized and light during the day and won't feel so exhausted. Think about how much more you will accomplish with this newly acquired energy.

M&M: Melon and Mint

Ingredients:

- ½ honeydew melon
- 1 bunch fresh mint
- 1 lemon
- 1 tsp raw honey

Directions:

Slice fresh honeydew and place in a bowl. Add fresh mint and a squeeze of lemon. Drizzle some raw honey on top, and viola! Start off warm, sunny days with a light melon salad.

Scrumptious Oats

Ingredients:

- 1 cup rolled oats
- 1 ripe banana
- ½ cup almond or rice milk
- 1 tsp raw honey
- 1 tsp ground flax (optional)

Directions:

Throw 1 cup of oats in bowl with water before you go to bed at night. Then when ready to eat in the morning, strain the water out of the oats and place them in a blender. Add 1 banana and ½ cup of almond milk and blend. Drizzle raw honey on top and sprinkle a dash of ground flax on top if you want to get some extra fiber, micronutrients, and omega-3 fatty acids.

The Perfect Date Raw Smoothie

Ingredients:

- 1 banana

- 3 dates
- 1 cup almond milk
- 1 tbsp raw honey
- 1 tbsp ground flax (optional)
- 1 tbsp hemp seeds (optional)

Directions:

Blend all ingredients until smooth. If you prefer cold you can add a few ice cubes or chill for 10 minutes.

Too Cool For School Cucumber Cleanse

Ingredients:

- 1 cucumber
- 1 sprig fresh mint
- 1 pear
- 1 lemon
- 1 slice ginger

Directions:

Blend all ingredients together and enjoy! You don't have to be at the spa to enjoy the wonderful benefits of cucumber. Although cucumbers are primarily composed of water, they are incredibly rich in nutrients and are a great source of vitamins C and A, silica, potassium, and magnesium. The skin is full of fiber and folic acid!

Kale Tales

- 6 leaves kale
- 1 pear
- 1 bunch fresh mint
- 1 handful wheatgrass

Directions:

Place all ingredients in the blender. Blend till smooth and enjoy!

The Hulk's Delight

- 1 bunch spinach
- 1 bunch kale
- 1 bunch collard greens
- 1 lemon

Directions:

Blend kale, spinach, and collard greens together. Pour in a glass and add a squeeze of lemon. This drink is definitely what I call a power drink. Forget heavy, sugary protein shakes. If you want to start your day off with a kick, this drink is a nutritional explosion! Spinach is rich in vitamins K, E, C, B2, B6, and B1, folic acid, magnesium, and iron! And kale alone is known as the most highly nutritional vegetable because it rich in carotenes, vitamins C, B1, B2, B6, and E, manganese, fiber, copper, iron, and calcium. These greens combined into one filling, delicious meal is a perfect way to start every day.

Granola Breakfast of Champions... and Hippies

- 1 cup sunflower seeds (soaked overnight till large and plump)
- 1 cup raw almonds (soaked overnight till large and plump)
- 1 cup golden raisins
- 2 tbsp hemp (optional)
- ½ tbsp dried coconut flakes

- 1 dash cinnamon
- 1 tsp raw honey

Directions:

Blend sunflower seeds, almonds, raisins, hemp, honey, and cinnamon together. Sprinkle dried coconut flakes on top and enjoy!

Berry Bliss

- ½ cup blueberries
- ½ cup strawberries
- ½ cup raspberries
- ½ cup blackberries
- 1 banana

Directions:

Blend all ingredients together. This drink is a perfect dose of antioxidants, being rich in flavonoids, vitamins C, E, B6, B2, and K, soluble fiber, insoluble fiber B1, iodine, folic acid, manganese, and niacin.

Pretty In Peach Summer Smoothie

- 1 ripe peach
- 1 banana
- 1 bunch of fresh mint

Directions:

Blend Ingredients together until smooth. Add ice. Garnish with fresh mint and enjoy!

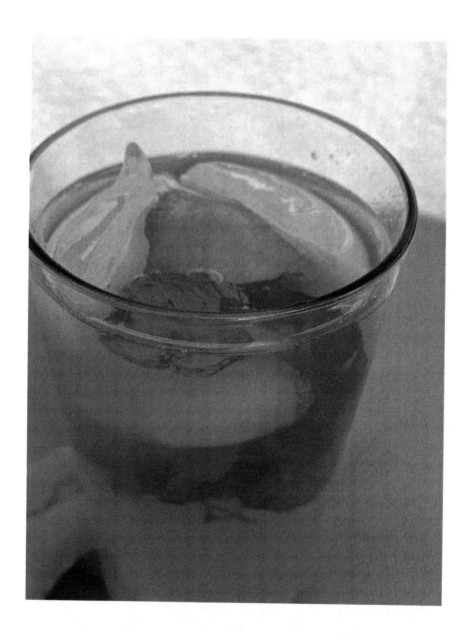

Snack Time

Here are a few healthier options for your favorite comfort-food snacks.

- Air-popped popcorn with a light drizzle of grape seed oil and a dash of Celtic sea salt
- Hummus and cucumbers
- Unsalted almond butter and raw honey on crisp apples or crunchy celery sticks
- Flax crackers
- Raw avocado
- Raw almonds (Store nuts in the refrigerator to maximize freshness.)
- Homemade trail mix: sunflower seeds, walnuts, pumpkin seeds, hemp, coconut flakes, raw cacao nibs, and a sprinkle of Celtic sea salt (All ingredients can be found at local health-food store.)

Lunch and Dinner: You Guessed It! More Fruits Veggies and Whole Grains

Note: You can add brown rice or quinoa to any of these recipes to make a more filling and satisfying meal.

Kick-Ass Kale Salad

Ingredients:
- 1 bunch organic kale (avoid greens that have yellowing leaves)
- 1 lemon
- 1tbsp grape seed oil
- ¼ cup raw walnuts

- ¼ cup golden raisins

Directions:

Rinse kale and rip into small pieces with your hands and put into a salad bowl. Add walnuts, raisins, and a splash of grape seed oil. Squeeze lemon on top and enjoy!

Tasty Taco...Margarita Not Included

Ingredients:

- 1 ripe avocado
- 1 lemon
- 1 dash cayenne pepper
- 1 bunch sprouts
- ¼ cup raw onions
- ½ ripe tomato
- ¼ cup goji berries or currants (optional)
- 1 collard green leaf or lettuce leaf (this will be the shell to wrap your taco in)

Directions:

Mash avocado in a bowl. Add cayenne pepper, lemon, and Celtic sea salt, and mix. Add sprouts, onions, tomato, and currants or Goji berries, and mix well. Then add a squeeze of lemon. Place this mixture in lettuce wrap, and viola! Guilt-free tacos—yum!

T and A: Tomato and Avocado Salad with Ginger Miso Dressing

Ingredients:

- 1 bunch fresh arugula
- 1 ripe avocado

- 1 fresh tomato
- 1 lemon
- 2 tbsp grape seed oil
- 1 slice ginger
- ½ cup fresh sprouts, micro greens, alfalfa sprouts, or whatever you like
- 1 tbsp white miso

Directions:

Place arugula, avocado, tomato, and sprouts in bowl. To make dressing, place fresh ginger, a squeeze of lemon, grape seed oil, and miso in the blender and mix till smooth. Pour over salad, and bon appetite!

Green Machine Salad

- 1 bunch kale
- 1 bunch spinach
- 1 bunch mixed greens
- ¼ cup shiitake mushrooms
- ¼ cup raw onions
- 1 heirloom tomato
- 1 lemon
- 2 tbsp olive oil

Or…for those of you who have a little extra time, here's a super yummy green dressing you can make.

Dressing:

- 1 bunch fresh mint
- 1 sprig parsley
- 1 lemon

- ½ cucumber

Directions:

Place washed kale, spinach, and mixed greens into a bowl. Add shiitake mushrooms, raw onions, and tomato. For fast and easy dressing, squeeze lemon over salad and add a sprinkle of olive oil. If you have more time, place mint, parsley, a squeeze of lemon, and cucumber in a blender. Mix until smooth and pour over salad. The mint and cucumber are wonderfully refreshing!

Cool As a Cucumber Soup

Ingredients:

- 1 cucumber
- 1 cup unsweetened almond milk
- 2 celery sticks
- 1 sprig dill
- 1 sprig mint
- 3 slices honeydew (optional)

Directions:

Slice cucumber into small pieces and toss in blender with almond milk, celery, mint, and honeydew. Blend until smooth. Place into a bowl and refrigerate for 3 hours until cold. Sprinkle dill on top.

Bloody Mary (Hangover Not Included)

Ingredients:

- 1 fresh red tomato
- 1 bunch cilantro
- 1 lemon

- 2 celery sticks
- ½ cucumber
- 1 sprig parsley
- 1 dash cayenne pepper

Directions:

Blend red tomato, cilantro, celery, cucumber and cayenne pepper—but don't blend too much. This soup is best when slightly chunky. Pour into a bowl, squeeze lemon on top, and sprinkle with parsley. Refrigerate for 3–4 hours before serving.

Guilt-Free Dessert

The Healthy Version of Chef's Chocolate Salty Balls From South Park

Ingredients

- 1 cup of raw ground almonds (you can get this at Trader Joe's)
- 5 dates (remove pits)
- 1 tablespoon of ground cinnamon
- 3/4 cups of raw cacao powder
- 1 sprinkle of Celtic sea salt
- 1 cup of shredded dried coconut flakes
- 1/3 cup of water

Directions:

Place almond flour, dates, cinnamon, cacao powder, Celtic sea salt, and water in a blender and mix well. Now here's the fun part. Light some candles, put on some Barry White and roll up your sleeves, cause its about to get messy. Get your palms wet and start rolling the batter into small bite sized balls. If your hands keep getting sticky, you can put a little coconut oil on your palms. (ladies ...you can take that one to the bank)

Note: Don't worry about making your balls perfect. In my opinion, misshapen balls tend to have more character! Lastly, dip and roll each ball into a bowl filled with shredded coconut flakes. Chill in the freezer for 2 hours. Then put them in your mouth and suck em !

Bashful Banana Pudding

Ingredients:
- 1 ripe banana
- ¼ cup unsweetened almond milk

Directions

Place banana in freezer and freeze overnight. Then place in banana in blender and add almond milk. Leave slightly chunky. Scoop into bowl and enjoy!

Cacao-Covered Strawberries

Ingredients:
- 1 package fresh, ripe, organic strawberries
- 2 tbsp raw cacao powder
- 1 tsp raw honey
- 1 tsp coconut oil
- ½ cup dried coconut flakes (optional)

Directions:

Mix cacao power, honey, and coconut oil in a bowl. Dip strawberries in chocolate and sprinkle with coconut flakes. Refrigerate for 2 hours and enjoy!

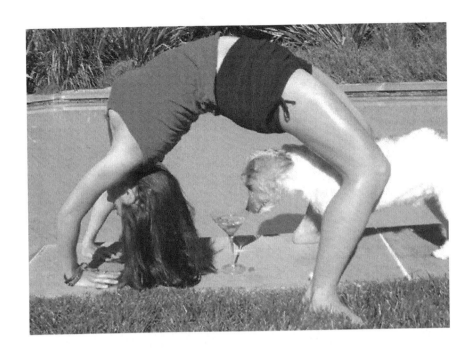

Addendum # 3:
Sample Daily Journal

"Knowing yourself is the beginning of all wisdom."
—Aristotle

Date: _____

Goals and Intentions for the Day

_____

_____
_____

_____

Daily Foods

BREAKFAST

_____

_____

_____

How Do I Feel?

_____

_____

_____

LUNCH

_____

_____

_____

How Do I Feel?

_____

_____

_____

DINNER

_____

_____

_____

How Do I Feel?

_____

_____

_____

Daily Exercise

_____

_____

_____

Addendum #3: Sample Daily Journal

How Do I Feel?

_____

_____

_____

Choices That Did Not Serve Me (Relationship, Nutrition, Ethics)

_____

_____

_____

I Am Grateful For:

_____

_____

_____

What Did I Do Today That Was Just for Me?

Endnotes

Chapter 1:

1. *Roger Williams Biochemical Individuality: The Key To Understanding What Shapes Your Health, The Basics of Genetotrophic Concept, September 11th 1998*

2. *D.Ornish, S.E Brown,L.W.Scherwitz, et al." Can Lifestyle Changes Reverse Coronary Heart Disease? Lancet 336(1990)*

3. *Ori Hofmekler's The Warrior Diet: Switch On Your Biological Powerhouse – For High Energy, Explosive Strength, and a Learner Harder Body, December 4th 2007*

4. *Michael Murray.N.D., The Encyclopedia of Healing Foods, pg 47 September 2005*

5. *Joshua Rosenthal, Integrative Nutrition: Feed Your Hunger For Health & Happiness, 2008*

Chapter 2:

1. *Dr. Kelley's contantly evolving workbook:* <u>*The ABCs of Natural Health*</u> *- The Natural Health Place, 1993*

2. *Joshua Rosenthal, Integrative Nutrition: Feed Your Hunger For Health & Happiness, 2008*

Chapter 4:

1. *Ori Hofmekler's The Warrior Diet: Switch On Your Biological Powerhouse – For High Energy, Explosive Strength, and a Learner Harder Body, December 4th 2007*

2. *Ori Hofmekler's The Warrior Diet: Switch On Your Biological Powerhouse – For High Energy, Explosive Strength, and a Learner Harder Body, December 4th 2007*

3. *Web MD Food-O-Meter: Food Calorie Calculator*-Find nutrition facts including calories, fat, carbohydrates, protein, sugar, fiber in over 37,000 foods and beverages. *http://www. webmd.com/diet/healthtool-food-calorie-counter, 2008*

4. *Rochester University Health Service (UHS) Health Promotion Office "Caloric Values of Alcoholic Beverages, 2011" http:// www.rochester.edu/uhs/healthtopics/Alcohol/caloricvalues.html*

Chapter 5:

1. Natasha Kyssa,The Simply Raw Living Foods Detox Manual. 2009

2. *Joshua Rosenthal, Integrative Nutrition: Feed Your Hunger For Health & Happiness, 2008 p 41-43*

3. *Joshua Rosenthal, Integrative Nutrition: Feed Your Hunger For Health & Happiness, 2008 p 67-68*

Chapter 6:

1. Dr.F. Batmanghelidj The Water Cure, 2008, http://www. watercure.com/

2. Tourles, Organic Body Care Recipes- 175 Homemade Herbal Formulas For Glowing Skin and a Vibrant Self, 2007,pg 21

3. *Joshua Rosenthal, Integrative Nutrition: Feed Your Hunger For Health & Happiness, 2008 p 221*

4. Michael Murray.N.D., *The Encyclopedia of Healing Foods , 2005 p 419-424*

Chapter 9:

1. *Joshua Rosenthal, Integrative Nutrition: Feed Your Hunger For Health & Happiness, 2008,p 41-43*

2. *Michael Murray.N.D., The Encyclopedia of Healing Foods , 2005 p 402-408*

3. *Michael Murray.N.D., The Encyclopedia of Healing Foods , 2005 p 349*

4. *Michael Murray.N.D., The Encyclopedia of Healing Foods , 2005 P 144-147*

5. *Michael Murray.N.D., The Encyclopedia of Healing Foods , 2005 p 217-218*

6. Kimberly Snyder" 5 Superfoods That Help Improve Your Memory."Kimberly Snyder's Health and Beauty Blog. 2012, http://www.kimberlysnyder.net/blog/2011/08/23/5-superfoods-that-improve-your-memory/

Chapter 10:

1. PBS Affluenza, hosted by Scott Simon, produced by John de Graaf and Vivia Boe, production of KCTS/Seattle and Oregon Public Broadcasting" http://www.pbs.org/kcts/affluenza/show/about.html

2. Ecodemia, Campus Environmental Stewardship at the Turn of the 21st Century: Lessons in Smart Management from Administrators, Staff, and Students by Julian Keniry http://www.nwf.org/nwf/campus/tools/publications/ecodemia

3. Brian Clark Howard, The Daily Green. Copyright © 2012 Hearst Communications, Inc., http://www.thedailygreen.com/green-homes/latest/recycling-symbols-plastics-460321

Made in the USA
Lexington, KY
26 February 2016